Self✛Test Nutrition Guide

How to improve your health and nutritional status through personalized tests

Dr. Cass Igram
Judy K. Gray, M.S.

Knowledge House
Buffalo Grove, Illinois

Printed by Cedar Graphics
311 Parsons Drive
Hiawatha, Iowa 52233-1458

For ordering information call 1-800-243-5242

ISBN: SB 0911119507
ISBN: HB 0911119515

Disclaimer

The contents of this book are not intended as a substitute for medical treatment. Individuals with serious medical illnesses should consult their physicians before beginning new treatments.

Table of Contents

Section I - The Nutritional Deficiency Tests

Section II - The Dietary Tests

Section III - Illnesses and Syndromes

Preface

Nutritional deficiency is a major cause of disease and ill health and not just in the Third World. The majority of individuals living in Westernized countries, such as the USA, Canada, Britain, and Germany, consume a considerable amount of processed food. As a result, nutritional deficiencies are relatively common. Unfortunately, Americans have been led to believe that they are immune to the occurrence of significant nutritional deficiencies. This belief has been perpetuated largely by the medical profession and dietitians. Simply put, the orthodox belief is that the typical American diet amply supplies an individual's nutritional needs. The use of the word "belief" is descriptive; the medical profession has lagged behind in providing proof for what it claims. The fact is research and clinical experience have thoroughly documented the existence of widespread nutritional imbalances and deficiencies in Americans. It is scientifically accepted that a wide range of mental and physical diseases are due exclusively to nutritional deficiencies. And why not? Tens of thousands of research articles are published every year, many in prominent medical journals, proving that *nutritional deficiencies and dietary imbalances play a greater role than any other factor in the genesis of ill health.*

Introduction

Wouldn't you like to know where you stand nutritionally? Optimal health is directly dependent upon how well we are nourished. Therefore, the crucial question is: Are our bodies deficient in specific nutrients, or are we getting all the vitamins, minerals, enzymes, fats, proteins, and carbo-hydrates we need?

The majority of people would like to learn as much as they can about their nutritional status. Students of nutrition are aware that the potential for achieving optimal health is largely dependent upon the quality of their diets as well as how thoroughly any existing nutritional deficiencies are determined and corrected.

The nutritional status of each person changes month by month, week by week, day by day, and even meal by meal. These variations are based upon such factors as social habits, medical care (such as drug therapy and/or surgery), exercise (or a lack of it), mental stress, and weather conditions. For instance, an individual who is exercising in hot weather and works up a sweat may rapidly become deficient in sodium and potassium, as well as vitamin C, despite being physically fit, while another person staying indoors in an air conditioned room might have all the vitamin C and sodium he/she needs. In contrast, an individual living in a cold climate is likely to become deficient in pantothenic acid, a nutrient crucial for maintaining the adrenal glands' response to cold weather. A surgical patient's nutritional status might be adequate prior to surgery, but afterwards he/she would likely become deficient in anti-stress nutrients such as vitamin C, pantothenic acid, riboflavin, zinc, selenium, magnesium, and amino acids. An individual taking cortisone readily becomes deficient in vitamin C and calcium, while someone who frequently consumes antibiotics will develop significant B-vitamin deficiencies.

Thus, in determining nutritional status it is important to realize that each person's circumstances are different and that there are numerous variables to consider. Additionally, the extent of the nutritional deficits that an individual suffers is often dictated by genetics. For instance, an inherited defect in B-6 metabolism may result in the need for as much as one hundred times the B-6 required by a normal individual.

Stress also determines nutritional requirements. For example, an individual experiencing mental duress, such as grief resulting from the loss of a loved one, marital discord, etc., may need double or triple the amount of vitamin C, zinc, and/or pantothenic acid compared to a person whose life is relatively stress-free. Pregnant and/or lactating women provide another illustration of the tremendous variation in nutritional requirements. They may require as much as five times the intake of certain nutrients as do women in the typical physiological state. However, despite these variables, the majority of individuals desire to know precisely what their nutritional status is so that corrective supplementation can be prescribed. Yet, most people lack a clear-cut method for making such determinations.

Certainly, it would seem, the medical profession is obligated to apply scientifically based methods for determining nutritional status, since for every disease there is a nutritional component. It is reasonable to presume that, in regard to nutritionally induced diseases, it is the physician's responsibility to become knowledgeable concerning the symptoms and consequences of nutritional deficiency. This is so that the appropriate diagnosis (or diagnoses) can be made. Further, it could be concluded that if an individual is suffering ill health as a result of nutritional deficiencies, his/her physician should be capable of performing various examinations, blood tests, and procedures in order to confirm precisely which nutritional deficiencies he/she has. This is a scientific approach to the diagnosis and treatment of disease and would help eliminate the guesswork which is so commonly applied in today's medical scene. It is unfortunate that in reality nothing could be further from the truth. Physicians possess little knowledge about nutritional diagnosis and know even less about nutritional prescription.

The complexity of the human body's nutritional chemistry can be compared to a puzzle. Each nutrient is like a piece of the puzzle, and the puzzle is never completed until the status of every nutrient is assessed. What's more, each disease can be regarded as a separate puzzle with its own unique "nutritional topography." Researchers have proven that every major disease has its own pattern of nutritional inadequacies. *It has also been determined that virtually every disease can be improved through diet.* Yet, the vast majority of today's physicians tend to minimize the crucial role played by nutritional deficiencies and/or dietary imbalances in the causation of disease. It is as if they have something better to offer—but they don't. Their only alternatives are drugs or similar therapies, which offer little hope for relief or cure.

Nutritional deficiencies are rampant in America today. True, it is rare to find a fulminant case of scurvy, starvation (i.e. kwashiorkor), or beriberi. However, such extremes of nutritional deficiency represent only the tip of the iceberg of the innumerable illnesses caused by nutritional deficits. Even so, certain severe nutritional deficiency diseases are far from rare. Rickets, which is due to vitamin D deficiency, is an example of a classical nutritional deficiency disease, and it is increasing in incidence even here in the United States. Hundreds of thousands of American children are afflicted with it, although black and inner city populations are particularly affected. People often make fun of "bow-legged"

4

children and/or teenagers. However, these children most likely have rickets, and no one realizes it.

A number of other serious problems can result from nutritional deficiency. Each year thousands of Americans are afflicted with a life-threatening disease which is, in fact, a manifestation of beriberi. It's called *Wernicke-Korsakoff's Psychosis,* and the victims are primarily alcoholics whose brains are destroyed as a result of alcohol induced thiamine deficiency. Untold millions of Americans suffer from another potentially life-threatening illness due almost exclusively to vitamin deficiency: pernicious anemia. This disease is the result of a deficiency of vitamin B-12. With this type of anemia there are usually plenty of red blood cells. However, the shape of the cells becomes distorted, and cells actually become enlarged. As a consequence of the genetic defects resulting from B-12 deficiency, the oxygen-carrying capacity of the red cells is significantly diminished. This leads to a variety of symptoms, including fatigue, lassitude, headaches, memory loss, depression, and mental confusion.

Perhaps the most common manifestations of pernicious anemia are the neuropsychiatric disorders which are associated with it. B-12 is involved in the synthesis of neurotransmitters, the chemicals which send messages within the brain and along the nerve sheaths. Recent research indicates that a growing body of individuals are developing psychiatric disorders, notably depression, paranoia, psychosis, and dementia, from poor vitamin B-12 nutriture. The elderly are particularly vulnerable, with some studies documenting low blood levels of B-12 in as many as one third of psychiatric patients over 55.

Thus, pernicious anemia, like scurvy, pellagra, or beriberi, is mainly a nutritional deficiency disease. In fact, virtually all types of anemia are caused by nutritional deficiency, with iron deficit being the usual missing link, although protein, B-vitamin, and other mineral deficiencies may also play a role.

5

In contrast, the medical profession primarily recommends drugs for the treatment of the majority of diseases, even those caused by nutritional disturbances. Aspirin is one prominent example. There is an intensive media blitz touting the "curative" value of aspirin for a wide range of diseases, including stroke, heart disease, hardening of the arteries, headaches, and even cancer. Lately, this drug has been touted in the medical journals as a prevention for digestive cancer. This recommendation can hardly be taken seriously, since aspirin *causes* a variety of digestive ailments. Despite this the medical profession continues to aggressively recommend aspirin. It's as if there is a global aspirin deficiency that is responsible for the maladies plaguing modern civilization. Ironically, medical literature supports the fact that aspirin causes a greater amount of disease than it cures and is, in fact, responsible for its own unique and potentially fatal disease: *Reye's Syndrome*. Further, several thousand individuals are admitted to hospitals every year in the United States alone as a result of aspirin toxicity; many die.

Because of its blood-thinning action, aspirin is the primary cause of acute bleeding from the stomach and/or intestine. Strokes (cerebral hemorrhage) can also result from aspirin consumption, since the blood vessel walls of the brain are weakened by it. In fact, the number of individuals who die every year as a result of aspirin induced internal bleeding numbers in the thousands.

Aspirin never was and never will be a "miracle cure." Those who believe that aspirin is the magic bullet should be aware that for every tablet consumed, the body loses several million molecules of vitamin C, beta carotene, selenium, vitamin E, vitamin K and essential fatty acids, since aspirin aggressively destroys these protective nutrients.

Nutritional deficiency is common in the United States. In some populations it is endemic, and in others it has become a rampant plague. For instance, all alcoholics are nutritionally deficient. Are there not millions of them?

6

The American public is obviously fraught with illness. In fact, the United States is the most disease-riddled society on earth. Cancer, heart disease, diabetes, stroke, arthritis, lupus, multiple sclerosis, Alzheimer's disease, Parkinsonism, psoriasis, colitis, hepatitis, obesity, depression, migraine headaches, and an assortment of other degenerative diseases afflict tens of millions. Additional untold millions suffer from vague complaints for which no diagnosis can be determined. These latter individuals are on the fringes, wavering between generalized ill health and frank disease. Thus, Americans are taking billions of drug tablets and capsules every year with good reason: they are sick and in pain.

Unfortunately, less than five percent of America's physicians receive training in the field of nutrition. Those who do take nutrition classes in medical school gain, at best, a cursory review. Today's physicians lack the skill necessary for diagnosing illnesses caused by nutritional deficiencies and often fail to recognize those caused by gross nutritional deficiency such as beriberi, scurvy, rickets, pernicious anemia, and pellagra. Doctors are simply unaware of the roles played by vitamin, mineral, protein, enzyme, and/or fatty acid deficiencies in the cause of generalized illness as well as gross disease. However, the primary reason for this "medical deficiency" is not merely the lack of training doctors receive; it seems that most physicians simply do not believe that poor or inadequate nutrition initiates disease. This is difficult to understand, since the medical journals are replete with data supporting the fact that nutritional deficiencies are a primary cause of chronic ill health. It is also despite the frequent nutrition-related endorsements by the National Cancer Institute, World Health Organization, and numerous other prestigious associations. Recently, the American Medical Association recognized the ineptness of medical professionals regarding nutritional awareness. They noted that the physicians of the future must discipline themselves to spend more time with their patients in the realm of nutritional and/or dietary advice.

Doctors appear to have an attitude problem concerning nutrition. Many feel that making a habit of giving out nutritional advice is below them and should be left to the dietitians. They feel that their time should be devoted to "real medicine," that is drug therapy, invasive diagnostics, and surgery. After all, how can dietary intervention compare in curative power to the potent drugs listed in the PDR?[1] How can improvements in diet and vitamin/mineral therapy rate with high-tech procedures such as laser surgery, angiography, angioplasty, and bypass surgery? How could nutritional medicines and herbal therapies possibly compare with chemotherapy and radiation? Right or wrong, this is how doctors think today.

The vast majority of medical professionals rely almost exclusively upon drugs and surgical procedures as the basis of treatment. These therapies are often described in medical circles as the "big guns," although they strike more like shotgun blasts than bull's-eye bullets. In contrast, research and clinical experience have proven that nutritional therapy *can* compare in effectiveness to orthodox medicine. Not only is it less toxic, but it is also often more specific and effective than comparable medical approaches. The recent discovery of the curative value of the Pacific Yew tree's effectiveness against ovarian cancer has proven that.

The typical nutritional recommendations given by doctors today are appalling to the sophisticated nutritionally oriented mind. Seeking advice from traditional doctors about nutrition is truly putting one's trust with the ignorant. It's like asking directions from someone who doesn't know the way; you are

---

1. *Physician's Desk Reference* is the standard manual used by doctors for delineating the type, usage, mechanism of action, and side effects of prescription medications.

likely to be steered onto the wrong avenue. Millions of Americans are advised by physicians and/or dietitians to eat margarine instead of butter, imitation cream instead of real cream, fake eggs instead of real eggs, synthetic cheese instead of real cheese, or artificial ice cream instead of real ice cream. We are told, "Stay away from avocados. They contain too much fat and cholesterol." Avocados do contain fat, but they have been wrongfully associated with cholesterol; they contain none. This is only one example of the nutritional nonsense continually being parlayed by so-called health authorities.

The low-fat milk theory is equally ludicrous. Americans are instructed to drink only skim milk (or 1% milk) and eat only skim milk cheese. How could highly processed milk products, as skimmed milk products are, be more health-enhancing than pure unprocessed milk[2] as it exists in Nature? The fact is as much as 75% of the vitamins and minerals in milk are found in the fat, and, thus, the process of skimming and adulterating milk leads to the destruction of much of its nutritional value. Recent research has confirmed this; studies conducted at the University of Massachusetts determined that skimmed milk products may be detrimental to health by increasing the risks for cataracts, cancer and heart disease.

Even though this is precisely the opposite of what the American public is being told about milk products, there is good substance for this alternative view. Milk is a whole food. Processing it by removing its fat disrupts its nutritional

---

2. "Pure unprocessed milk" is also referred to in the remainder of this book as "whole milk" or "fresh milk." Dietary recommendations for milk should be interpreted to mean whole unprocessed milk. Unprocessed means milk not pasteurized or homogenized, in other words "raw" milk. Unfortunately, certified raw milk is available in only a few states, notably California and Oregon. Unhomogenized (but pasteurized) goat's milk is available in numerous farm states, including California, Iowa, Illinois, and Wisconsin.

value and makes it less digestible. Here is why. Milk naturally contains sugar in the form of lactose. Chemically, lactose is a *disaccharide*, meaning that it is composed of two sugar molecules bound together by chemical bonds. One of these sugars, galactose, can be highly irritating if separated from the milk sugar bonds. That is precisely why fat naturally occurs in milk. It acts as a sealant, protecting the lactose from being destroyed and, thus, preventing the release of the highly irritating galactose. When the fat is skimmed from the milk, the lactose is vulnerable to oxidation, and this results in the release of free galactose. Apparently, the potential toxicity from the free galactose is such that if enough of it accumulates in the body, tissue damage may result. This at least partially explains the research finding that people who regularly consume skimmed milk products instead of those made from whole milk have as much as a threefold higher risk for certain diseases, notably cancer and heart disease.

Currently, beans are being touted as an exceptional food source. However, they fare poorly as a source of quality nutrition when compared to traditional protein sources such as meats, fish, eggs, and milk products. What's more, bean allergy is common, and the major culprits are kidney beans, pinto beans, and mung beans. Legumes, which are related to the bean family, are a richer source of protein, minerals, and vitamins than beans. Yet, here again, allergy is a significant problem, as tens of millions of Americans are intolerant to the various foods of the legume family, particularly peanuts, lentils, split peas, soy beans, and/or chick peas. However, for those who can tolerate them, legumes are an excellent source of nutrients and are usually preferable to beans. In fact, beans are one of the most indigestible of all foods, because they contain natural chemicals called *lectins*. These compounds frequently provoke severe allergic intolerances and gastrointestinal distress. Beans cannot be regarded as an adequate replacement for the super-nutrition foods that nutritionists are attempting to displace by them.

Imitation or "laboratory" food is a modern food scheme. Synthetic food is always inferior to real food. There is no nutritional value in coffee creamer: no viable vitamins, fatty acids, or minerals. Instead, its list of ingredients includes corn syrup, hydrogenated vegetable oils, food dyes, sulfites, and MSG. In contrast, real cream contains numerous nutrients and is usually free of additives. The only justifiable reason for replacing real cream with coffee creamer is in the case of butter-fat or milk allergy, and even then it would be more nutritionally sound to "drink it black" than to add imitation cream. The same is true of ice cream; if you are going to indulge in it, for heaven's sake eat the real thing with the least amount of additives.

Artificial eggs also fail to bring significant nutritional value to the table. After all, what is the nutritional value of food dyes, hydrogenated oils, artificial flavors, and processed egg whites compared to real eggs? Eggs are loaded with nutrients and are one of Nature's richest sources of protein, vitamin A, folic acid, lecithin, riboflavin, vitamin E, biotin, chromium, iron, and, yes, cholesterol. Compare this list of critical nutrients contained in real eggs with the ingredients found in artificial eggs, which are devoid of virtually all of these aforementioned nutrients. In fact, there simply is no comparison. It is truly appalling that such a senseless recommendation as replacing real eggs with egg substitutes could be made despite its glaringly erroneous nature. Yet, millions of Americans continue to follow such advice, literally like so many lambs being herded by their shepherds to slaughter.

A good rule is to always opt for the foods synthesized by Nature over those synthesized by man. Even as noxious as refined sugar is, it is perhaps less damaging to consume it rather than the sugar substitutes, which are nothing more than synthetic chemicals. The human body has the capacity to digest sugar, since it is a naturally occurring substance. This is not so with the artificial sweeteners, such as NutraSweet and saccharin, both of which are produced from petro-chemical waste products. The safety of these sweeteners for human consumption has never been proven. On the contrary, evidence is accumulating that artificial sweeteners are toxic even in relatively small amounts. Saccharin, which is a coal tar derivative, has long been suspected of being a carcinogen and has been linked to the cause of bladder cancer. NutraSweet causes a wide range of symptoms and illnesses, including temporary and/or permanent blindness, nerve disorders, behavioral disorders, digestive disturbances, and migraine headaches.

There are a host of other fake foods and synthetic food additives, far more than can be listed in these pages. All are devoid of nutritional value and, in fact, detract from nutritional status by destroying nutrients and/or impairing their absorption. Here are a few examples. Synthetic iron destroys vitamin E, vitamin C, and beta carotene. Brominating agents, such as those used to fumigate fruit and bleach flour, destroy vitamin C, vitamin E, beta carotene, riboflavin, pantothenic acid, potassium, and selenium. Sulfites oxidize vitamin C, molybdenum, riboflavin, and folic acid. Food dyes inactivate vitamin B-6, folic acid, and vitamin C. Ethylene glycol, the main constituent of antifreeze and a relatively common food additive, destroys vitamins A, C, E, and the mineral selenium. The preservatives BHT and BHA destroy vitamins A, C, and E. EDTA, a chelating agent, prevents the absorption of minerals such as zinc, calcium, and magnesium. Pesticides, residues of which are found in virtually all commercial foods, inactivate vitamin C, vitamin E, B-6, digestive enzymes, and selenium. Chlorine inactivates thiamine and destroys vitamins A, C, and E. Chlorine is found in foods packed in water as well as in all municipal water supplies. Fluoride, which is found in most municipal water supplies, destroys vitamins B-1, C, E, and beta carotene and disrupts the function of virtually all human enzymes.

To make matters worse, our food, even if fresh and unprocessed, contains less nutrients than ever before in American history. Commercial farming practices are the main culprits. Prior to the turn of the century all foods grown in this country were "organic." This means they were grown on virgin soil without the use of toxic chemicals. In that age the health-giving qualities of food were regarded as more important than economic concerns. In contrast, the primary goal of modern farmers is to achieve a high yield per acre. The nutritional quality of food is rarely an issue. As a result, Americans survive on food which appears to be normal, but in actuality is nutritionally defective.

Over the past 60 years farmers have dumped untold tons of chemicals in the form of fertilizers, pesticides, fungicides, and herbicides onto the soil. This practice has damaged the soil to such a degree that there are far less nutrients in it compared to the original virgin state. Thus, food grown on depleted soil absorbs a reduced amount of nutrients. What's more, agricultural chemicals bind what few minerals are left in the soil, making them unavailable for absorption into the crops. That is one of the major reasons there is a virtual epidemic of trace mineral deficiency in the USA. As a consequence, ill health is on the rise. Mineral deficiency may be manifested by common symptoms, such as fatigue or depression, or may ultimately cause serious and/or life-threatening diseases.

Many farmers are aware of this critical connection between trace minerals and health. The lack of single trace minerals in the soil can cause a significant reduction in crop yield and, in the extreme, may cause crop failure. Animals readily become mineral deficient if they are fed primarily commercially grown crops. In fact, cattle can be so damaged by a lack of certain minerals that they may become crippled or may even drop dead en masse. Newborn animals are particularly vulnerable to sudden death from nutritional deficiency. Symptoms of mineral deficiency in cattle include hoof and mouth disease, arthritis, belly bloating, diarrhea, weight loss, skin eruptions, lung infections, bone deformities, hair loss, infertility, and loss of appetite.

Pesticides and herbicides bind minerals by an action known as chelation, making them unavailable to plants. Commercial fertilizers also bind minerals. Some examples of the adverse effects of farm chemicals on the soil are as follows:

Chemical	**Soil Nutrient**
Lime	Binds zinc and manganese and impedes copper intake
Nitrogenous fertilizers	Impair copper absorption into plants
Phosphates	Create excess absorption of molybdenum and impair calcium uptake
Potash (potassium)	Causes boron deficiency in plants
Pesticides/herbicides	Impair the absorption of all essential minerals

The importance of this data is emphasized by the fact that 99% of the food grown in the United States is produced on soil fertilized with commercial fertilizers.

Soil erosion has also contributed to a decline in mineral levels. Thus, it is no surprise that researchers have discovered trace mineral deficiencies in the soil of virtually every state in the country. For instance, some 30 states have suboptimal soil zinc levels. Virtually all have reduced magnesium levels. Few if any states have adequate soil levels of selenium, cobalt, and/or copper. Thus, the food is mineral deficient even before it is fumigated, brominated, chlorinated, refined, sweetened, waxed, stored, or cooked. For these reasons virtually every American whose diet consists of commercial food is deficient in at least one of the trace minerals and usually several of them.

Trace minerals are the essence of life and are of even greater import than the vitamins. While they are given the designation of "trace," compared to the quantity of vitamins normally found in the body, they are abundant. They are the essence of life, because they modulate cellular function by stimulating and controlling the rate of cellular reactions. It is through the enzymes that minerals exert this effect, since minerals are the spark plugs which catalyze them. Most human enzymes contain a mineral fixed within amino acids. Take zinc, for example. It is an integral component of hundreds of human enzymes. As a result, zinc is essential for the stimulation of millions of enzymatic reactions every fraction of each second. In fact, such a large number of enzymes are zinc dependent that researchers have been unable to fully quantify them. Other minerals heavily involved in enzymatic functions include magnesium, selenium, copper, manganese, molybdenum, and potassium.

The human body thrives on minerals. Unfortunately, Americans eat few mineral-rich foods. Instead they consume large quantities of mineral-depleted foods such as white flour products (including pasta), white rice, refined corn products, refined sugar, commercially grown fresh produce, and canned produce.

The American public is interested in nutrition, and this interest is growing exponentially every year. People are aware that what they eat has a major influence upon how they feel. They are beginning to realize that the traditional American diet isn't all that it is touted to be. They are starting to feel the difference—the improved energy and enhanced well-being that results from eating right.

An insignificant minority of American physicians practice nutritional medicine, that is the treatment of disease with vitamins, minerals, enzymes, herbs, fatty acids, and other natural substances. Thus, perhaps the greatest "deficiency" in America today is that of the nutritional physician. This is an immense problem, since health—and the loss of it—is a complexity, one which should be addressed by professionals, not the public. Yet, most nutritionally oriented people know that top-notch nutritional physicians are hard to locate. This problem is most extreme in small cities and towns. However, there is a similar shortage in many major cities. Where these nutritional doctors do exist, the population densities are astronomically high. A city the size of Dallas might have five or ten such physicians, while supporting several hundred traditional doctors.

For physicians who are interested in nutrition, this book could serve as a boon. That is because it can be used as a historical guide for the evaluation of nutritional illness. However, it was written equally for lay people, who, in contrast to the majority of physicians, are convinced of the health-enhancing value of nutrition. It is also written for those who find it difficult to access nutritionally oriented physicians.

Does this mean that this book is a diagnostic manual, that people can read it and determine precisely what deficiencies or illnesses they have? Not at all. It is simply a guidebook to provide clues for what might be wrong. Only a licensed medical professional can establish a diagnosis: books can't. Diagnostic testing is the primary method for procuring a diagnosis, and obviously this can only be achieved by a licensed physician. Additionally, a thorough history and physical exam are crucial elements for making a diagnosis. This quiz book is an information source which provides an enjoyable method for learning more about your body. Treat it that way, and you will benefit from it. Use it to make a diagnosis, and you could do yourself harm. Diagnoses are made in health professionals' offices and in hospitals. However, this book can help you be more aware of potentially dangerous symptoms. If you are experiencing any symptoms or signs of serious disease, consult your physician.

It is easy to understand why the American public has developed a growing interest in nutritional therapy. Many people have a certain degree of disillusionment with the medical profession. Drug therapy has become sort of out of vogue. Millions of people refuse to take medicines, primarily because they are wary of their toxic effects. Surgery is no longer regarded as an absolute cure of choice. Invasive diagnostic testing is often scary, and the side effects are numerous and potentially serious.

The medical profession has failed to find a cure for common degenerative diseases such as heart disease, arthritis, diabetes, lupus, Alzheimer's disease, and/or cancer. Thus, the incidence of these diseases rises every year. However, what may be of greater concern is the fact that certain diseases previously regarded as rare are dramatically rising in occurrence. The connective tissue diseases are one example. These diseases include lupus, fibromyalgia, fibromyositis, dermatomyositis, scleroderma, rheumatoid arthritis, and osteoarthritis. Nutritional therapy can produce significant improvement in these diseases and certainly is of greater value than the drugs currently used to treat them.

Perhaps of greatest concern is the rising incidence of infectious diseases. Children are besieged by episodes of upper respiratory, intestinal and ear infections. Adults suffer with bouts of colds, flu, food poisoning, kidney/bladder infections, and/or intestinal infections as well as pneumonia. The sexually transmitted diseases are no longer simply a source of embarrassment or chronic illness; they are outright killers and will soon be listed among the top five causes of death in this country. A frightening and recent development is the outbreak of drug-resistant tuberculosis infections. Tuberculosis is also on the rise in children, despite

17

immunizations. This is largely because of outbreaks of drug-resistant strains of TB in hospitals. Furthermore, recent outbreaks have been traced to sites which place untold millions at risk: the air systems/filters in jet airlines. In fact, the circumstance is so ominous that researchers claim all of the advances made in TB treatment over the past century will be reversed in a mere twenty years or less. An additional concern is the Chronic Fatigue Syndrome, a disease which primarily affects adults. This debilitating condition has been correlated to infections by viruses and parasites, although the exact cause remains unknown.

How to Get the Most Out of this Book

The purpose of this book is to educate individuals about nutrition, that is their own personal nutrition. Particular emphasis is placed upon the determination of each individual's nutritional status. At the end of each exam information regarding corrective nutritional supplementation and dietary advice is provided. Those who are willing to change dietary and social habits that impair good nutrition will receive the greatest benefits from this book.

Millions of Americans are "addicted" to certain foods and find the thought of change overwhelming. The fact is the American diet is permeated with addictive substances; caffeine, MSG, sugar, white flour, cocoa, vanilla bean, food dyes, artificial sweeteners, and alcohol are prominent examples. It is not surprising that many Americans find themselves so attached to their dietary and social habits that they feel helplessly and hopelessly addicted. This is certainly true of the majority of coffee, chocolate, cigarette, sugar, and alcohol "junkies." Yet, despite this dilemma, habit restructuring is as simple as this: you can change—*if you want to*.

Heredity and environmental factors play critical roles in influencing the capacity for individuals to readily alter

nutritional habits. Family members often share deficiencies.
This may be due to genetics, but it may also be the result of
environmental factors.   Parents who smoke are constantly
polluting their children's lungs with cigarette smoke.   Not
only does the smoke cause nutritional depletion, but it also
increases the youths' risks for a variety of diseases, including
heart disease, cancer, lung disease, asthma, and immune
deficiency. What's more, many children inherit the pattern of
deficiencies seen in smokers as a consequence of being
exposed to the residues of cigarette smoke while they are in
the womb or during their formative years.

Children have little choice but to adhere to the dietary
norms of their parents and grandparents.   If the parents
and/or grandparents are sugar addicts, so too will the children
become addicted. However, as bizarre as it may seem, some
parents carefully watch their diets while they feed their
children all manner of junk food ranging from hot dogs,
hamburgers and French fries to Twinkies. Here is the point:
all family members should take the quizzes. See if a pattern
develops.   Then, the entire family can follow a nutritional
rebuilding program.   It is much easier to adhere to new
dietary habits if everyone joins together in the effort.

When taking the tests, a question may arise regarding the
past or present: Which is most important as far as analyzing
the results? The score that you register right now, which is
representative of your current lifestyle, is the most meaning-
ful one. However, it is also of value to test how you would
have scored previously, for instance, as a child, teenager, or
perhaps as you lived five or ten years ago. This will provide
the most comprehensive picture of your nutritional status and
will help determine the extent of your nutritional needs.

Family members should assist each other in the disciplin-
ary action required for changing from a processed and junk
food diet to the consumption of nutrient-rich whole foods. In
other words, they should work together as a team.

Inevitably, temptations will overcome discipline and some people will falter. Encourage such individuals to give it their best effort. The benefits from eating right are immense and well worth the endeavor. Better health, improved energy, increased vigor, improved appearance, healthier skin, disease prevention, and, in some instances, the stalling of the aging process are all likely consequences of the effort to eat right.

In order to evaluate your progress, document your symptoms, past and present, in a looseleaf notebook. Make sure you record the date of the entry and label each group of symptoms under the nutrient deficiency category. The following entries from a typical symptom log is based upon the upcoming vitamin B-1 deficiency test. Obviously, in this example the individual's symptoms have improved:

Date	Symptoms — B1
08/12/93	2. nervousness 7. chronic constipation 13. irritability
11/12/93	7. constipation (occasional)

After you make dietary improvements and take the appropriate nutritional supplements, it is wise to retest yourself to see if the symptoms have diminished. Do this at least every three months until your symptoms are reduced to your satisfaction. Then check your status periodically—once or twice a year—to maintain a general awareness of your nutritional well being. Remember, good health is your greatest treasure.

Section I

The Nutritional Deficiency Tests

Vitamin B-1 (Thiamine)

The existence of B-vitamins was conceived less than 100 years ago. In the early 1900s Casimir Funk, a Polish biochemist, proposed the existence of certain dietary substances required in trace amounts for the prevention of diseases that were the plague of that era, notably beriberi and pellagra. Researchers later (1915) determined that food contained both water and fat soluble vitamins. Using egg yolks as the raw material, they extracted the vitamins and named the fatty fraction "fat soluble A" and coined the name for the water fraction, "water soluble B." Eventually, chemists were able to isolate two of the vitamins, thiamine and riboflavin, from the water soluble fractions. Once isolated, the chemical formulas of the individual vitamins were identified, and, ultimately, they were synthesized.

However, to their surprise, researchers found something highly intriguing. The purified and/or synthetic compounds were considerably less effective than the original crude extracts made from foods. Apparently a number of other unknown factors worked in concert with the known vitamins. The chemists' intensive search for these unknown factors led to the discovery of the remaining B-vitamins: niacin, folic acid, vitamin B-12, biotin, pantothenic acid, and pyridoxine. Future research will likely reveal yet-to-be-discovered fractions.

Thiamine deficiency is common in the United States. This is despite the fortification of processed foods, notably breads and cereals, with the nutrient. Gross deficiency of thiamine causes a condition known as *polyneuritis*. This is defined as inflammation of the nerve sheaths throughout the body. Obviously, thiamine is required for the normal functioning of the nerves. It is no surprise that this important B-vitamin is known as the *morale vitamin*. In fact, mood changes, depression, and/or other mental symptoms are early signs of its deficiency.

Anyone who believes that thiamine deficiency in America is rare should consider the following study. Volunteers were placed on a standard American menu of bread, processed cereals, well-done beef, potatoes, white rice, gelatin, egg whites, sugar, cocoa, skimmed milk products, canned fruits, canned vegetables, and coffee. The diet was supplemented with every nutrient except thiamine. In addition, the volunteers were given thiamine-deficient brewer's yeast. This was done to ensure that any symptoms that might occur could be assigned exclusively to thiamine deficiency. In fact, the diet was so well supplemented that in all respects, with the exception of thiamine nutriture, it was superior to that eaten by the majority of Americans. According to the researchers, "All the volunteers became irritable, depressed, quarrelsome, uncooperative and...fearful that some misfortune awaited them. Two became so agitated that they felt life was no longer worth living and threatened suicide. In part, this could be attributed to weakness, in part to inability to concentrate, confusion, and uncertainty of memory..."

There are a number of reasons that thiamine deficiency is common in America and other civilized societies. First, the so-called civilized diet is largely composed of highly processed and refined foods, while thiamine occurs naturally in large quantities only in wholesome unprocessed foods. Such foods include whole grains, particularly the germ and bran fractions, fresh organ meats, peanuts, and soybeans. Secondly, naturally occurring thiamine is a rather delicate compound and is readily destroyed by cooking. Losses during storage may also be significant, and fluorescent light negatively affects it. What's more, thiamine is inactivated by chlorine, and, thus, people who wash and/or cook their food with chlorinated water or, more importantly, drink, bathe, or swim in chlorinated water are likely to become thiamine deficient.

One way to prevent thiamine loss while cooking is to add acidic substances, such as lemon juice or vinegar, to the

23

cooking medium. Apparently, acids stabilize the thiamine molecule, preventing heat-induced destruction. Thus, thiamine depletion is reduced when preparing recipes naturally high in acid such as spaghetti sauce, tomato soup, and fish in lemon sauce.

Thiamine is absorbed chiefly from the upper part of the small intestine, i.e. the duodenum. Thus, diseases of that region, for instance, duodenal ulcer, pancreatitis and giardiasis (a parasitic infestation of the small bowel), greatly hamper thiamine absorption and lead to its deficiency.

People who regularly drink black tea often develop thiamine deficiency, since tea contains compounds which block thiamine absorption. Raw sea foods, such as sushi, herring, oysters, and lox, can induce thiamine deficiency, since these foods contain a thiamine antagonist called *thiaminase*. In actuality, this is an enzyme which attacks the thiamine molecules, splitting them in half. Individuals who suffer from liver disease of any type (hepatitis, cirrhosis of the liver, Gilbert's disease) are vulnerable for developing severe thiamine deficiency. Additionally, alcohol destroys thiamine. One or more drinks per day is enough to induce severe thiamine deficiency. For chronic alcoholics, particularly those who drink a pint or more of alcohol daily, thiamine deficiency can become so extreme as to result in irreparable nerve and brain damage. The function of all brain cells is thiamine dependent; it is no wonder that thiamine-deficient alcoholics develop a wide range of mental symptoms, including depression, memory loss, agitation, violent behavior, and frank psychosis.

To perform the thiamine test and all subsequent tests, add the total number of positive responses and match your score with the mild, moderate, severe, or extreme deficiency categories. Each response is worth one point unless otherwise indicated. It is desirable to keep a record of your deficiencies and check to see if the symptoms decrease with dietary intervention and supplementation.

Which of these apply to you?

1. depression and/or anxiety
2. nervousness
3. sugar intolerance
4. lack of appetite or excessive appetite
5. vague chest pains and/or shortness of breath
6. irregular heartbeat
7. chronic constipation
8. indigestion
9. intolerance to protein-rich foods such as meats, soybeans, milk products, and fish
10. leg cramps after exercising
11. agitation
12. chronic fatigue
13. irritability
14. sleep apnea
15. anger
16. fears and/or paranoia
17. excessively rapid heartbeat with mild or moderate exercise
18. rapid resting heartbeat (80 beats or greater per minute)
19. heaviness and/or weakness of the arms or legs
20. burning and/or numbness of the arms, hands, feet, and/or toes
21. personality changes
22. heartburn
23. swelling of the extremities
24. bloating after eating
25. stomach aches and/or pain
26. attention deficit (i.e. short attention span)
27. mental dullness and/or poor concentration
28. loss of strength
29. vulnerability to insect bites, particularly fleas and mosquitoes
30. bed wetting

31. temper tantrums and/or violent behavior
32. craving for sugar and/or other sweets
33. apathy or feeling of impending doom
34. eye fibrillations (twitches)
35. lack of sensation for urination (lack of urination)
36. loss of muscle tissue in arms and/or legs
37. premenstrual depression
38. painful menses
39. noise sensitivity
40. rapidly aging skin
41. nausea and/or vomiting
42. cold hands, ears, and feet
43. hypotension (low blood pressure)
44. headache
45. insomnia
46. excessive sweating
47. abdominal pain
48. inability to maintain weight
49. foot and wrist drop
50. tendency to stumble while walking or climbing stairs
51. clumsiness
52. sleep walking
53. nightmares
54. chronic swelling of the lymph nodes
55. Do you have an abnormally slow heart rate?
56. Do you have a history of retinal bleeding?
57. Do you have a history of bulimia?
58. Do you regularly consume alcoholic beverages (one or more drinks per day)?
59. Do you consume black or iced tea on a daily basis?
60. Do you consume raw fish on a daily or weekly basis?
61. Do you have chronic backaches which are unresponsive to traditional therapies?
62. Do you drink two or more cups of coffee on a daily basis?
63. Are you emotionally unstable?

64. Are you quarrelsome or argumentative?
65. Do you have a low pain tolerance?
66. Do you have a phobia of the sensation of creatures (insects) crawling on your skin?
67. Do you have an enlarged heart (cardiomyopathy)?
68. Have you had a portion of your stomach or intestines removed, or have you undergone stomach stapling?
69. Do you adhere to a high carbohydrate diet?

Your Score _____

1 to 9 points *Mild thiamine deficiency:* Even mild thiamine deficiency can result in significant symptoms and predispose individuals to certain diseases. Correct this by eating thiamine-rich foods (Appendix A) and supplementing the diet with rice polishings (or *Nutri-Sense*, see page 301), which is one of the richest food sources known. Consume 2 heaping tablespoons of rice polishings mixed in milk, water, or juice daily. Additionally, alcohol and refined sugar destroy thiamine, so their intake must be reduced or eliminated.

10 to 22 points *Moderate thiamine deficiency:* Aggressive correction of moderate thiamine deficiency will help prevent future health problems or resolve existing ones, since chronic thiamine deficit often results in a variety of physical and mental derangements. Eat large helpings of thiamine-rich foods and consume 2 to 3 heaping tablespoons of rice polishings morning and night. Additionally, take a multiple vitamin containing thiamine. Avoid the thiamine destroyers, a category which includes raw fish, green or black tea, coffee, refined sugar, chlorinated water, and alcohol.

23 to 33 points *Severe thiamine deficiency:* A variety of potentially serious medical conditions may result from prolonged thiamine deficiency. These conditions include malabsorption, underactive or overactive thyroid, dementia,

depression, anxiety, congestive heart failure, immune defects, heart rhythm disturbances, hypoglycemia and/or diabetes, and even beriberi. If you have any of these diseases, it is likely that you are thiamine deficient. Correct this deficiency by fortifying baked goods and cereals with rice polishings. In addition, take 3 heaping tablespoons of rice polishings three times daily mixed in juice, water, or milk. Thiamine supplements are also indicated. However, the typical type of thiamine found in vitamin pills, thiamine hydrochloride, is poorly absorbed. A superior type is fat-soluble thiamine, which is found in a supplement called *Allithiamine*. Take 100 mg (i.e. mg = one milligram = 0.001 gram) of Allithiamine morning and night.

34 and above   *Extreme thiamine deficiency:* Warning— physiological derangement, as well as internal organ damage, is imminent if tissue thiamine levels continue to decline. The nervous system, including the brain, is particularly vulnerable and can be damaged irreparably unless the deficiency is corrected promptly. Take supplemental thiamine, preferably in the form of Allithiamine, a highly absorbable fat-soluble form of thiamine. The initial dosage should be 300 mg three times daily. After 60 days of this therapy reduce the dosage to 200 mg three times daily. Additionally, fortify foods and cereals with rice bran and/or polishings and mix 4 heaping tablespoons of rice polishings in juice, water, or milk and drink this mixture morning, noon, and night. If symptoms persist, see your doctor.

Severe thiamine deficiency can be corrected by injections of this B-vitamin. However, there is a word of caution: intravenous/intramuscular thiamine has been associated with toxicity, including severe allergic reactions. Thus, taking thiamine orally is safer than injections. In fact, evidence is accumulating that the fat-soluble thiamine is the safest form of all. Additionally, it is better assimilated. A study was recently performed comparing the absorption of oral doses of fat-soluble thiamine with the absorption of injectable thiamine. The researchers were amazed to find the blood levels were consistently higher with the oral dosage of Allithiamine than with the injectable form.

With the exception of alcoholics suffering from *delirium tremens*, correction of the thiamine deficiency with oral doses should suffice. For the alcoholic with extreme thiamine deficiency, the next drink might be the fatal one, since life-threatening cardiac and/or neurological symptoms may develop as a result of alcohol-induced thiamine deficiency. Thus, alcoholics who score high on this exam must stop drinking alcoholic beverages immediately. However, they should do so only while under a doctor's care to avoid the *delirium tremens*, which is potentially fatal. *Note:* Allithiamine and *Nutri-Sense* Drink Mix may be purchased from Nutritional Supplement Service, phone (800) 243-5242.

Vitamin B-2 (Riboflavin)

As early as the 19th century, scientists noticed that certain foods possessed a yellow-green fluorescent pigment. They found this pigment in a wide range of foods, including milk, eggs, almonds, organ meats, and vegetables. Because of their fluorescent nature, these pigments were called "flavins," which ultimately led to the naming of riboflavin. Originally, this B-vitamin was called "lactoflavin," since its presence was first observed in milk.

Riboflavin deficiency may be induced by poor nutrition, high consumption of sugar, severe infections, surgery, birth control pills, and/or malabsorption. Other factors which may create a deficiency include lack of stomach acid, antibiotic usage, diuretics, and mental stress. Additionally, malabsorption, high protein intake, faulty lipid metabolism, acute injuries, pregnancy, and lactation all increase the need for riboflavin. The riboflavin content of foods is dependent upon a variety of factors. Farm fresh (unheated, unprocessed) foods offer the highest amounts. Riboflavin losses may be as high as 90% in commercial foods, including "fresh" produce. That is because riboflavin is a highly unstable substance. It is readily destroyed by light, particularly fluorescent light. For example, milk stored in plastic jugs and glass containers loses the majority of its riboflavin content by the time it is consumed.

One of riboflavin's most critical functions relates to oxygen metabolism. Riboflavin accelerates the capacity of the lungs to remove oxygen from the air. In addition, it aids in the transfer of blood oxygen into the cells and is also crucial for the utilization of oxygen at the cellular level. Sufficient riboflavin in the lungs helps protect the body from the ill effects of air pollution.

Top sources of riboflavin include organ meats, muscle meats, eggs, almonds, caviar and, to a lesser degree, dark green leafy vegetables. Starchy foods, such as beans, grains, and potatoes, are generally poor sources of this vitamin. Additionally, riboflavin is more readily absorbed from meat than from vegetable sources. Riboflavin may well be one of the most difficult of all vitamins to procure in the diet because of its instability and rarity in the food supply.

Which of these apply to you?

1. inflamed and/or swollen tongue
2. bloodshot eyes or conjunctivitis
3. cracks at the corners of the mouth
4. depression
5. dizziness
6. burning and/or itching of the eyes
7. blurred vision
8. sensitivity of the eyes to light (photophobia)
9. eczema
10. lips which are constantly chapped

11. cholesterol and/or whitehead-like deposits on the face
12. crusting of the eyelids (granulated eyelids)
13. wrinkles radiating from lips towards nose and cheeks
14. poor wound healing
15. excessive tearing of the eyes
16. insomnia
17. unusually red or whitish lips
18. decreased hand grip strength
19. digestive disturbances
20. mood swings
21. nervousness
22. abnormal or excessive appetite
23. a feeling of "sand" under the eyelids
24. chronic acne
25. loss in the width (fullness) of the upper lip
26. fatigue
27. sores around and/or in the mouth
28. lack of concentration
29. irritable colon
30. dandruff
31. painful tongue
32. eye fatigue
33. chronic sinus problems
34. eyelid spasms/twitching
35. myopia (nearsightedness)
36. greasy facial skin, especially on the nose
37. lips which are swollen, inflamed, and/or crack easily
38. scaly greasy lesions on scrotum or vulva
39. tendency to walk or stand with feet turned inward
40. visible tiny red blood vessels about the nose or on the cheeks
41. tongue which is cherry red or reddish blue in color
42. roughening or thickening of the skin on the nose
43. Do you use chewing tobacco?
44. Do you smoke cigarettes (1/2 pack or more per day)?
45. Do you consume alcohol on a regular basis?

46. Do you take birth control pills or have you in the past taken birth control pills for a prolonged time (five or more years)?
47. Do you suffer from chronic lung disease?
48. Do you urinate frequently or with excessive volume?
49. Have you had your duodenum removed, or are you suffering from duodenal ulcer?
50. Are you taking cholesterol-lowering medications?
51. Do you suffer from retinal detachment or retinitis?
52. Do you have macular degeneration?
53. Do you suffer from corneal ulcers?
54. Do you consume refined sugars on a daily or weekly basis?
55. Do you have chronic dermatitis and/or dermatitis due to light or metal sensitivity?
56. Are you a vegetarian?
57. Do you regularly take diuretics?
58. Do you take antibiotics on a daily, weekly, or monthly basis?
59. Do you have a history of cataracts?
60. Do you have anemia that has failed to respond to iron therapy?
61. Do you sunburn easily, or do you develop rashes from sun exposure?
62. Are you constantly rubbing your eyes?
63. Do you have bald spots (atrophy) on your tongue?

Your Score ____

1 to 9 points *Mild riboflavin deficiency:* Riboflavin is a tightly controlled nutrient in terms of tissue storage/losses, since it is firmly bound within the cells. However, even a modest reduction in tissue stores results in cellular dysfunction. Mild riboflavin deficiency may be corrected by taking a multiple vitamin containing riboflavin and by curtailing the consumption of refined sugar and alcohol, both of

which destroy this nutrient. Add hefty portions of riboflavin-rich foods to the diet.

10 to 21 points *Moderate riboflavin deficiency:* At this stage individuals may suffer from certain medical conditions, including myopia, astigmatism, alopecia, and/or growth impairment. Correct the deficiency by taking a multiple vitamin containing riboflavin, plus a B-complex tablet containing 25 or 50 mg of riboflavin. Additionally, include riboflavin-rich foods such as organic meats (especially liver), lean red meat, and fresh dark green leafy vegetables.

22 to 34 points *Severe riboflavin deficiency:* Significant impairment of the function of the cells and internal organs, especially the liver, may occur at this level of deficiency. An aggressive program should be instituted for replenishing tissue riboflavin stores. Create riboflavin-rich menus. In addition to a multiple vitamin, take a B-complex tablet containing at least 50 mg of riboflavin twice daily. Take also desiccated buffalo liver (4 capsules 3 times daily), the richest natural source of riboflavin. Strictly avoid refined sugar and alcohol.

35 and above *Extreme riboflavin deficiency:* If the tissue riboflavin content falls to a critical level, the system responsible for the production of cellular energy fails to function properly. Furthermore, prolonged extreme riboflavin deficiency may result in permanent damage of the skin, nerves, and/or internal organs. The skin, hair, and eyes are particularly vulnerable. Diseases such as cataracts, macular degeneration, retinal detachment, eczema, alopecia, and premature aging are likely to occur. Correct the deficiency by taking 100 mg of riboflavin morning and night. Additionally, take 6 capsules of desiccated buffalo liver 3 times daily. Also take a multiple vitamin containing all the B-vitamins and load up on riboflavin-rich foods.

Vitamin B-3 (Niacin)

The need for niacin was first establish as a consequence of the discovery of a severe disease. This disease, called pellagra or "rough skin," was originally described by a Spanish physician during the 18th century. Pellagra was well known to American physicians of the early 20th century, since it was at that time one of the leading causes of illness and death. However, pellagra was unique compared to most of the diseases of that era. It is exclusively a disease of poor diet, the consequence of the refinement of whole grains, corn, and rice. Pellagra is a sort of final proof, however crude and destructive, that "man cannot live on bread alone"—white bread, that is.

Niacin is readily absorbed throughout most of the small intestine. However, mental stress, alcohol/drug abuse, prescription drugs, and processed foods all cause niacin depletion. Since little niacin is stored in the body, a deficiency may rapidly occur. As a result, tissue levels must be continually replenished.

Niacin is essential for fat metabolism, transport, and digestion. It helps mobilize fat from adipose tissue so that it can be burned as energy. It prevents the buildup of cholesterol within the liver and arteries and is a natural cholesterol-lowering agent. Niacin is also involved in the synthesis of the protective fatty covering of the nerves, the myelin sheath.

Niacin exists in nature in several forms. The most well researched are nicotinic acid and niacinamide. The amino acid tryptophan may be regarded as a form of niacin, since, if niacin stores are depleted, it is readily converted into the vitamin. Thus, a diet rich in tryptophan may provide sufficient niacin, even though the diet is low in the actual vitamin. This is why corn-rich diets induce niacin deficiency, since corn is low in both niacin and tryptophan. Additionally, small amounts of niacin are synthesized in the intestines by normal bacterial flora. Top sources of tryptophan include red meats, poultry, fish, rabbit, cheese, eggs, and sesame seeds. Excellent sources of niacin include organ meats, fresh muscle meats, rice polishings, eggs, and cheeses.

Which of these apply to you?

1. lack of appetite
2. muscular weakness
3. indigestion
4. loss of memory and/or mental acuity
5. depression
6. patches of dry scaly skin (rough skin)
7. chronic diarrhea
8. chronic fatigue
9. bad breath
10. emotional instability
11. insomnia
12. chronic headaches
13. vague abdominal pains
14. dementia/senility
15. dermatitis, especially of hands and/or face
16. sore tongue and/or mouth
17. rectal irritation
18. irritability and/or anxiety
19. psychotic behavior
20. mood swings
21. chronic joint pain and stiffness (arthritis)
22. black coloration of the tongue
23. rough patches of skin in the mouth
24. large brown blotches on the skin
25. Do you consume, on average, one or more alcoholic beverages per day?
26. Is your cholesterol level greater than 230 (untreated)?
27. Do you have a history of cocaine, crack, or heroin abuse?

28. Do you have a history of manic-depressive syndrome or schizophrenia?
29. Do you consume refined sugar on a daily or weekly basis?
30. Do you have a duodenal ulcer, or have you had your duodenum removed?
31. Do you consume corn as a major part of your diet (Mexicans, vegetarians, etc.)?
32. Do you have low stomach acid (hypochlorhydria)?
33. Do you have undigested food in the stool?
34. Do you have neurological disease manifested by a loss of sensation, nerve inflammation, and/or nerve damage?
35. Do you have bald spots on the tongue?
36. Do you have deep fissures (trenches) in the tongue?
37. Do you have dermatitis/inflammation of the scrotum?

Your Score _____

1 to 7 points *Mild niacin deficiency:* Mental disturbances, such as depression and memory loss, are the most likely consequences of mild niacin deficiency. Fatigue is also a common symptom. Correct this by taking a multiple vitamin tablet containing niacin and by consuming niacin-rich foods, particularly brown rice, tuna, trout, salmon, halibut, peanut butter, poultry, and liver. Additionally, take 2 heaping tablespoons of rice polishings daily.

8 to 14 points *Moderate niacin deficiency:* This degree of niacin deficiency is usually the consequence of a high sugar diet. Refined grains and alcohol are other major niacin destroyers. Niacin is of crucial importance in energy metabolism. Without it, the body's fuels—sugars, starches, and fats—cannot be utilized by the cells, that is burned as fuel. The result is the accumulation of sugars and/or fats within the blood stream. This is the reason that niacin has been utilized as a heart drug. In pharmaceutical dosages it

36

helps reduce abnormally high blood levels of cholesterol and triglycerides. To correct the niacin deficit, take a B-complex tablet containing niacin twice daily. Additionally, consume 3 heaping tablespoons of rice polishings twice daily. Supplement the diet with niacin-rich foods and avoid refined sugars, white flour, refined corn products, white rice, and alcohol.

15 and above *Severe niacin deficiency:* Warning—severe niacin deficiency is associated with an increased incidence of a variety of diseases, including high cholesterol, diabetes, heart disease, dementia, hypertension, arteriosclerosis, and arthritis. To correct this deficit, take a B-complex capsule or tablet morning and night along with 250 mg of niacin. In addition, take 4 to 6 heaping tablespoons of rice polishings three or four times daily and consume hefty helpings of niacin-rich foods. Strictly avoid all alcoholic beverages and refined sugars.

Vitamin B-5 (Pantothenic Acid)

Pantothenic acid was discovered in 1933 by the noted American biochemist Roger Williams. Dr. Williams found that animals deprived of vitamin B-5 developed a variety of degenerative diseases and eventually died. After many years of research on pantothenic acid, Dr. Williams concluded that the vitamin was commonly deficient in the American diet. In his words, "it is wishful thinking to suppose that people always get enough (from their diets)." Further, Dr. Williams provided convincing data that humans require as much as twice the pantothenic acid as animals. What's more, he clearly documented the heightened need for B-5 in individuals suffering from constant psychological stress. Thus, it is no surprise that soon after he published his research, pantothenic acid became known as the "anti-stress vitamin."

Pantothenic acid should also be nicknamed "the power vitamin." That is because a deficiency of pantothenic acid results in weakness and/or fatigue, and supplementation with it usually leads to an immediate increase in vitality and strength. It makes sense that pantothenic acid would have this effect. It is required for the synthesis of adrenal hormones, and these hormones are responsible for the human body's ability to cope with the normal stresses of existence and the abnormal ones as well.

The adrenal glands produce dozens of hormones, each of which is an essential component of the stress-coping mechanism. These hormones are also involved in the maintenance of normal body functions, such as salt and water retention, blood sugar regulation, anti-inflammatory activity, calcium and magnesium metabolism, libido, and immune activation.

Stress rapidly depletes tissue stores of pantothenic acid. Without adequate amounts of this vitamin, the stress-induced deficiency of adrenal hormones becomes extreme. A severe deficiency of adrenal hormones may lead to a potentially fatal disease known as *Addison's disease*. More commonly, individuals suffer from the debilitating but rarely fatal condition called *subclinical Addison's disease*. This condition results in such a wide range of symptoms that it is often underdiagnosed by physicians. This is unfortunate, since untold millions of Americans suffer from this debilitating condition.

Millions of Americans suffer from extreme and prolonged psychological stress. It is crucial to realize that the invaluable and life-preserving adrenal hormones are "used up" by stress. People who have endured prolonged stress are usually severely deficient in both pantothenic acid and adrenal hormones. What's more, prolonged stress, as might occur from grieving, chronic health problems, and/or marital discord, can damage the adrenal glands, but only if a deficiency of pantothenic acid exists. This illustrates how crucial it is to maintain adequate tissue stores of the vitamin.

Regular supplementation with pantothenic acid can help reverse stress-induced adrenal damage.

One particularly amazing feature of pantothenic acid is that a deficiency can cause symptoms to develop rather rapidly. Usually, it takes several months or perhaps years for a deficiency of a nutrient to surface in the form of symptoms and/or ailments. In contrast, vitamin B-5 deficiency may cause symptoms to occur within days. Researchers discovered that a whole catalog of illnesses and symptoms resulted when pantothenic acid was selectively removed from the diet of human volunteers. Perhaps the most dominating finding was the damage that occurs to the adrenal glands as a result of pantothenic acid deficiency. The researchers discovered that this damage was particularly acute if the adrenal glands were already severely stressed. Stress combined with pantothenic acid deficiency resulted in cell death within the glands. As a result, the ability of the glands to produce adrenal hormones was severely impaired. However, when the diet was supplemented with pantothenic acid, the damage was prevented and the function returned to normal.

Unfortunately, pantothenic acid is found in large amounts in relatively few foods. Top sources include organ meats, egg yolks, muscle meats, soybean flour, and royal jelly. Fruits, pasta, vegetables, and most beans are devoid of pantothenic acid. Thus, strict vegetarians frequently develop B-5 deficiencies.

Which of these apply to you?

1. chronic fatigue
2. fall asleep more easily sitting up
3. insomnia
4. bloating and/or distension after eating
5. rapid pounding of heart/pulse on exertion
6. burning feet and/or heels
7. hard pebble-like stools

8. chronic constipation
9. vague abdominal pains
10. nervousness
11. mood swings
12. anxiety and/or panic attacks
13. depression
14. extreme weakness
15. muscle cramps, especially cramps in the feet or toes
16. quarrelsome or hot-tempered behavior
17. low blood pressure
18. susceptibility to infections, especially sore throats
19. patchy hair loss (alopecia)
20. lack of coordination
21. faintness or fainting spells (blackouts)
22. crying spells
23. nausea and/or vomiting
24. eczema and/or psoriasis
25. jumpiness and/or shakiness
26. noise sensitivity
27. headaches
28. food allergies
29. sensitivity to chemicals
30. infrequent urination
31. compulsive behavior
32. inability to cope with stress
33. excessive sweating of palms and feet
34. impaired memory
35. pains in the lower neck and upper back
36. receding gums
37. vague abdominal pain
38. lack of appetite
39. restless leg syndrome (constant motion of legs at night)
40. bruxism (grinding of the teeth and clenching of the jaw at night)

41. sleep apnea
42. sleepiness during the day
43. agitation and/or temper tantrums
44. Do you take cortisone and/or use cortisone creams?
45. Have you been under severe stress recently?
46. Do you have a history of severe allergic disease such as hives, eczema, and/or asthma?
47. Do you consume alcohol on a regular basis (one or more drinks per day)?
48. Do you have chronic joint pain?
49. Do you have a history of TMJ syndrome?
50. Do you suffer from frequent outbreaks of herpes (cold sores, genital herpes, shingles)?
51. Do you have chronic pain in the mid to lower back that is described as "kidney pain?"
52. Is your hair turning gray prematurely?
53. Do you suffer from diabetes or hypoglycemia?
54. Do you have a history of gout attacks?
55. Do you fall asleep spontaneously or uncontrollably during the day (narcolepsy)?

Your Score _____

0 to 11 points *Mild pantothenic acid deficiency:* Take 100 mg of pantothenic acid three times daily. Minimize the consumption of refined sugars and grains.

12 to 22 points *Moderate pantothenic acid deficiency:* Take 500 mg three times daily. Increase the consumption of foods rich in pantothenic acid, including royal jelly, bee pollen, organic liver, and fresh meats. Follow a low sugar and starch diet. Reduce the consumption of alcohol and avoid caffeine.

23 to 34 points *Severe pantothenic acid deficiency:* Take 1,000 mg three times daily. Avoid refined sugar and severely restrict alcohol intake. Take one teaspoon of royal jelly with

breakfast and dinner. Increase the consumption of foods rich in protein and natural fats and reduce your carbohydrate intake. Carbohydrates, particularly refined ones, stress the adrenal glands and increase the demand for pantothenic acid. Curtail the consumption of all dietary sources of refined sugar, white flour, caffeine, and alcohol.

35 and above   *Extreme pantothenic acid deficiency:* Warning—extreme debilitation, that is fatigue, weakness, mental derangement, and chronic pain, are likely to develop at this level of deficiency. Prolonged extreme B-5 deficiency may result in the onset of degenerative disease, including arthritis, asthma, immunodeficiency, lupus, heart rhythm disturbances, hypoglycemia, and diabetes. Follow the afore-mentioned dietary advice, and take 1,000 mg of pantothenic acid four times daily. If you scored above 42 points, your dosage of pantothenic acid is 2,000 mg 4 times daily (or 2,500 mg three times daily). Ideally, spread out the dosage as much as possible, since this ensures constant stimulation of adrenal steroid synthesis. Additionally, take one teaspoon of royal jelly three times daily; royal jelly is the richest known naturally occurring source of pantothenic acid. Vitamins A, C, E, and B-6, as well as the minerals selenium, chromium, and magnesium, are extra-important, since they help conserve pantothenic acid. Be sure to take them on a daily basis. Avoid all foods containing refined sugars, and curtail the consumption of alcoholic beverages. Alcohol destroys pantothenic acid. Caffeine weakens the adrenal glands and aggravates the B-5 deficiency state by causing the loss of this nutrient through the urine. All sources of caffeine and caffeine-like substances, such as cocoa, coffee, tea, soft drinks and vanilla bean, should be eliminated from the diet.

Vitamin B-6 (Pyridoxine)

Recent scientific studies indicate that the potential for pyridoxine deficiency in America has been grossly under-estimated. As many as 60% of Americans may be severely deficient in the vitamin.

This widespread B-6 deficiency has potentially serious consequences. That is because B-6 controls a broad range of physiological processes, including enzyme synthesis, fat and carbohydrate metabolism, protein digestion and metabolism, hormone production, and neurotransmitter synthesis. However, its most critical role relates to protein synthesis. The production of virtually all proteins within the human body, of which there are thousands, is dependent upon B-6. Additionally, B-6 is required for the synthesis of the genetic material—DNA and RNA—and, thus, it is an essential nutrient for the reproduction of all cells. What's more, the health of the immune system is dependent upon B-6. According to Dr. Phillip L. White, former director of the A.M.A's Department of Food and Nutrition, vitamin B-6 "is needed for the production of antibodies as part of the body's immune response." He also notes that it is required for the synthesis of hemoglobin. Both antibodies and hemoglobin are proteins. In addition, research by Axelrod proved that, of all B-vitamins, pyridoxine is the most crucial one for enhancing immune function.

Perhaps of equal importance as its role in protein synthesis is the function of B-6 in fatty acid synthesis. Without B-6, fatty acid metabolism comes to a screeching halt. We can live without protein for weeks or even months (although not without some ill consequences), but a complete deficiency of essential fatty acids, which may occur in association with severe B-6 deficiency, can rapidly lead to life-threatening diseases. (See essential fatty acid deficiency quiz, pages 169-174.)

Vitamin B-6 is an invaluable aid in the treatment of a variety of illnesses, including carpal tunnel syndrome, high blood pressure, diabetes, depression, anxiety, and insomnia. Like vitamin C, entire books have been dedicated to elaborating upon the medicinal values of B-6. An example is *The Doctor Who Looked at Hands*, by John Ellis, M.D. He describes the close relation between B-6 deficiency and heart disease. Dr. Ellis provides convincing evidence that the nerves of the heart, as well as the heart muscle itself, become damaged in the event of B-6 deficiency. He also stresses the interrelation between B-6 deficiency and joint disease, describing how the administration of B-6, either by mouth or preferably via injection, rapidly eliminated joint pain and swelling in individuals suffering from arthritis. Further, according to Dr. Ellis the seemingly epidemic problem of fluid retention is due largely to B-6 deficiency. Millions of Americans suffer from this pervasive problem, and women are most vulnerable. Fluid can accumulate in the face, within or under the eyelids, in the fingers and hands, over the sacrum, in the ankles, over the abdomen, and in the lower legs. Premenstrual fluid retention is a distressing symptom, and women can gain as much as eight pounds during a single menstrual cycle. Dr. Ellis describes how hundreds of his patients have been relieved of this annoying condition by taking 50 to 100 mg of vitamin B-6 daily.[3]

The digestion and absorption of protein is dependent upon adequate supplies of vitamin B-6. Additionally, this vitamin is required for the formation of a variety of highly specialized nervous system proteins called neurotransmitters. These compounds include adrenalin, noradrenalin, serotonin, GABA, and tryptophan. Other functions of vitamin B-6 include RNA

---

3. **Caution**: Megadoses of B-6 should be consumed only under a doctor's care. Evidence exists that dosages of B-6 above 100 mg per day may cause temporary and, in some instances, permanent nerve damage.

synthesis, hormone synthesis, antibody synthesis, and white blood cell formation.

B-6 is a natural anti-depressant. It is used as an invaluable adjunct in the treatment of chronic mental disturbances. As little as 50 mg per day may produce significant mood elevation. Studies have shown that it can even be helpful in the treatment of notoriously difficult to cure mental disorders, including retardation, anxiety, schizophrenia, mania, sleep disorders, and/or autism. Additionally, B-6 is of value in the treatment of epilepsy, particularly the types that occur in infants and young children. Epilepsy usually responds to megadoses of B-6, and the dosages are often so high that they should be taken only while under a physician's care.

Vitamin B-6 deficiency has been associated with peripheral nerve disorders such as diabetic neuropathy, sciatica, paraesthesia, and carpal tunnel syndrome. Carpal tunnel syndrome may well be the number one complaint in the workplace today. It's touted as being due solely to the repetitive movement of the hands and arms. While it is largely a mechanical problem, poor diet often initiates the abnormality by inducing B-6 deficiency. However, giving vitamin B-6 alone may not solve this problem. That is because the metabolism of B-6 within nerve fibers is controlled by thyroid hormone. Therefore, defective thyroid function, despite the presence of adequate B-6 levels, can lead to carpal tunnel syndrome. When treated with natural thyroid medication and the appropriate nutrients, especially B-6, there is improvement in the majority of cases—without surgery.

Only a small amount of B-6 is stored in the body, and it is rapidly depleted by stress. Many drugs destroy it, and the list includes aspirin, high blood pressure medicines, cortisone, laxatives, birth control pills, Dilantin, and antibiotics. Additionally, fluorescent light inactivates vitamin B-6. Thus, much of the food in the supermarket is depleted of B-6 by the time it is consumed. Pyridoxine is water

45

soluble, so much of it is lost when vegetables and other foods are boiled. The following are typical examples of B-6 losses in processed foods:

white flour: 80%
white rice: 85%
canned juice: 40%
canned vegetables: 60-90%
preserved meats: 70%
canned fruits: 50-70%

Of the foods rich in B-6 only poultry and fish are commonly consumed in the American diet. Other excellent food sources include rice bran, brown rice, wheat bran, sunflower seeds, soybeans, and organ meats.

Which of these apply to you?

1. inability to digest protein
2. indigestion and/or heartburn
3. nausea and/or vomiting
4. acne, particularly whiteheads
5. constipation
6. chronic fatigue and/or exhaustion
7. insomnia
8. mood swings
9. fluid retention
10. nervousness and/or agitation
11. low blood pressure
12. convulsions and/or epilepsy
13. confusion
14. depression
15. seborrheic dermatitis, especially of the face or nose
16. reddened tongue and/or smooth tongue
17. muscular weakness
18. oily hair

19. loss of texture and/or shine of hair
20. premature aging of facial skin
21. irritability
22. bad breath
23. swelling of the face, abdomen, and/or extremities during menses
24. dryness and/or scaling behind the ears
25. poor concentration (or attention deficit disorder in children)
26. dry patches of skin on the face and/or scaly facial skin
27. dry eyes
28. blurred vision
29. excessively dry hair
30. night-time leg cramps
31. tooth decay
32. tendency to cry easily
33. hair loss
34. lack of dreams or dream recall
35. lips which are constantly chapped
36. enlarged facial pores
37. Are you highly sensitive to MSG?
38. Have you ever been diagnosed with protein in the urine?
39. Do you have an abnormally high cholesterol?
40. Do you have a history of kidney stone formation?
41. Does chronic depression, psychosis, schizophrenia, and/or mania run in the family?
42. Do you regularly take diuretics?
43. Do you regularly consume birth control pills?
44. Do you regularly consume alcoholic beverages (4 or more drinks per week)?
45. Do you regularly take cortisone?
46. Do you currently take antibiotics on a daily, weekly, or monthly basis?
47. Do you have a history of melanoma?
48. Does your skin crack open easily, especially during the winter or as a result of stress?

49. Do you gain weight during or prior to your menstrual period?
50. Do you have a history of carpal tunnel syndrome?
51. Do you have a history of mitral valve prolapse?

Your Score ____

1 to 9 points *Mild B-6 deficiency:* Vitamin B-6 is a nutrient of such vast importance that even a minimal deficiency may produce symptoms. Perhaps the most common result of mild B-6 deficit is a lack of dream recall or no dreams at all. Mental disturbances, such as short-term memory loss and/or depression, may also result. Correct this deficiency by taking a B-complex tablet morning and night and by supplementing the diet with B-6-rich foods.

10 to 20 points *Moderate B-6 deficiency:* At this stage individuals become vulnerable for the development of illnesses due to B-6 deficiency. Such illnesses include depression, anxiety, epilepsy, kidney stones, melanoma, diabetes, PMS, carpal tunnel syndrome, eczema, and heart disease. To correct this deficiency, take a B-complex tablet twice daily in addition to 25 mg of B-6 twice daily. Reduce the B-6 dosage by one half after 2 months.

21 to 34 points *Severe B-6 deficiency:* Severe B-6 deficit can result in a variety of symptoms and/or illnesses. Aggressive treatment should include a B-complex tablet taken twice daily along with an additional 50 mg of B-6. Supplement the diet with large helpings of foods rich in B-6, including tuna, salmon, liver, white meat of fowl, nuts, halibut, and bananas. Reduce the total B-6 dosage to 50 mg once daily after 2 months.

35 and above *Extreme B-6 deficiency:* Extreme B-6 deficit may precipitate a variety of illnesses. B-6 is required for the

synthesis of a variety of proteins which are essential to life. Impaired protein synthesis/digestion may contribute to the onset of asthma, migraine headaches, hives, and other allergy-induced diseases. Musculoskeletal conditions, such as fibromyalgia, fibromyositis, back pain, neck pain, carpal tunnel syndrome, and arthritis, also have been correlated with B-6 deficiency and/or impaired protein digestion. Additionally, since B-6 is involved in kidney function, abnormalities involving this system, such as kidney stones, kidney infections, premenstrual edema, peripheral edema, and congestive heart failure, may occur. The brain and nervous system require B-6 for the production of neurotransmitters, for instance, serotonin, acetylcholine, and norepinephrine. Thus, it is no surprise that when tissue levels of B-6 drop to a critical point, depression, anxiety, psychosis, mania, insomnia, and even convulsions (epilepsy) may result. Follow the same recommendations as listed previously, and take 100 mg of B-6 three times daily. Reduce this dosage to 100 mg daily after 2 months.[4]

Folic Acid

It is difficult to conceive of a nutrient of greater importance than folic acid. It is involved either directly or indirectly in virtually every chemical reaction occurring within the body.

---

4. **Warning**: Studies have shown that dosages of B-6 in excess of 100 mg per day may be associated with nerve damage. Individuals who consume megadoses of B-6 must do so with caution. Be sure to take a B-complex supplement every day if you are taking 50 mg or more of B-6. Take the recommended megadoses (100 mg or more daily) for only as long as it takes to cause symptom improvement, then reduce the dosage to a maintenance level. Dosages above 500 mg per day should be consumed only under a doctor's care. On the positive side, B-6 is infinitely safer than aspirin, Motrin, Tylenol, and similar over-the-counter drugs.

That is because folic acid controls the very basis of human existence: the growth of cells. All cells depend upon this vitamin for their growth and regeneration. Thus, there is no life without folic acid.

Folic acid deficiency is alarmingly common in the USA, with all age groups being adversely affected. Perhaps of greatest concern are the results of recent scientific studies indicating that as many as 90% of teenagers are consuming less than the RDA of folic acid in their diets. Certain high risk groups, particularly blacks, fare even worse. For instance, an article in the *Journal of the American Dietetic Association* revealed that nearly 100% of black youths in certain schools in Mississippi received less than one-half the RDA for this crucial nutrient. Add to this the fact that many teenagers maintain habits that cause the destruction of folic acid, and it is easy to comprehend why this deficiency is so widespread and how tissue levels of the vitamin may become dangerously low. Agents which deplete and/or destroy folic acid include alcohol (as little as one drink per day may severely reduce tissue folic acid levels), cigarette smoking, chewing tobacco, stress, antibiotics, aspirin, marijuana, and hard drugs.

The term folic acid was originally derived from the Latin word *folium,* which is also the basis of the English term foliage. Thus, the origin of the word folic acid was due to the fact that this nutrient is commonly found in green edible plants. Actually, it was first isolated from spinach. Research in the 1940s determined that folic acid helped cure two serious diseases: megaloblastic anemia of pregnancy and malabsorptive syndrome (tropical sprue).

Researchers have discovered that folic acid can be utilized as a potent therapy for a variety of degenerative diseases. These diseases include arthritis, cancer (particularly pre-cancerous lesions), alcoholism, anemia, anxiety, depression, pyorrhea, PMS, gout, irritable bowel syndrome, Crohn's disease, ulcerative colitis, heart disease, macular degeneration, cataracts, and atherosclerosis. One notable study was performed to test the ability of folic acid to reverse arterial disease in the elderly. Subjects were given 5.0 to 7.5 mg of folic acid daily. As a result over 90% exhibited improved circulation, plus there was an unexpected benefit: enhanced vision. This was attributed to the localized improvement in circulation within the blood vessels of the eyes. In other words, folic acid helped reverse the aging-induced arterial degeneration which typically occurs within the tiny capillaries that feed the retina. Other studies document how megadoses of folic acid can reverse pre-cancerous lesions of the oral mucosa, lungs, intestines, and uterine cervix.

Top sources of folic acid include organ meats, yeast, chicken, soybeans, rice bran, dark green leafy vegetables, lean beef, veal, eggs, and whole grains. Organically grown foods contain a greater concentration of folates than those grown by commercial farming methods. Pesticides and herbicides destroy folic acid, as do fumigants, which are used to spray fresh produce. Additionally, folic acid is highly sensitive to light, and prolonged storage of food under fluorescent light may lead to a dramatic decline in folate levels. Cooking also destroys this vitamin, and as much as 95% may be lost during the preparation of food. The signs are easy to read: Americans are not getting enough folic acid to maintain optimal health, and some individuals are getting so little as to predispose them to a variety of potentially serious diseases.

Which of these apply to you?

1. hangnails
2. chronic diarrhea
3. chronic constipation
4. delayed wound healing
5. muscle cramps
6. lack of appetite

7. heartburn and/or indigestion
8. inflammation and/or soreness of the tongue
9. cracks at the corners of the mouth
10. lips which are constantly chapped
11. breathing difficulties
12. insomnia
13. chronic fatigue
14. muscular weakness
15. paranoia
16. depression
17. memory loss
18. growth impairment
19. dry and/or brittle hair
20. slow growing nails and/or hair
21. mouth sores (canker sores)
22. chronic cough (especially smoker's cough)
23. diminished resistance to infection
24. receding and/or bleeding gums
25. chronic gum infections (pyorrhea)
26. Do you eat most of your food canned, cooked, boiled, or fried?
27. Do you have a history of intestinal parasitic and/or fungal infection?
28. Do you have celiac disease and/or wheat allergy?
29. Do you have a history of abnormal pap smears, cervical dysplasia, and/or cervical cancer?
30. Do you have a history of chronic anemia unresponsive to iron or B-12 therapy?
31. Do you have chronic mental illness such as psychosis, anxiety-depression, mania, or schizophrenia?
32. Have you had one or more children with birth defects (spina bifida, etc.)?
33. Do you drink one or more alcoholic beverages daily?
34. Do you smoke cigarettes heavily (one-third pack or more per day), or have you smoked heavily in the past for over five years?

35. Do you use chewing tobacco?
36. Do you smoke cigars or pipes?
37. Do you regularly take birth control pills?
38. Do you take antibiotics on a daily, weekly, or monthly basis?
39. Do you take Dilantin?
40. Do you consume antacids on a daily or weekly basis?
41. Do you take Tagamet or Zantac on a daily or weekly basis?
42. Do you take one or more aspirin daily?
43. Are you on the drug Methotrexate and/or are you undergoing chemotherapy?
44. Are you undergoing radiation therapy or have you undergone such therapy recently?
45. Do you have gout?
46. Have you been diagnosed as having reduced protein (globulin, creatinine, or BUN) or low uric acid levels in your blood?

Your Score _____

1 to 9 points *Mild folic acid deficiency:* Folic acid is such a crucial nutrient that the functioning of the human body is impaired even in mild deficiency states. To correct the condition, take at least 400 mcg of folic acid daily and increase the consumption of folic acid-rich foods.

10 to 19 points *Moderate folic acid deficiency:* Take a B-complex tablet in addition to 5 mg of folic acid. Eat dark green leafy vegetables on a regular basis. Fresh meats are also an excellent source of folic acid, and to achieve optimal benefits, eat red meat medium rare. Be sure to consume the juices of the meat; this is where most of the folic acid is found. Other excellent sources include brown rice and dark green leafy vegetables. Avoid refined sugar, alcohol, white flour, and caffeine, all of which deplete or destroy folic acid.

20 to 29 points *Severe folic acid deficiency:* Symptoms of folic acid deficiency rapidly dissipate once cellular levels are replenished. Treat this condition aggressively by taking 10 mg of folic acid daily. Follow the aforementioned dietary advice; in addition, avoid all drugs which destroy folic acid, particularly aspirin. Try the Folic Acid Shake (see the recipe section).

30 and above *Extreme folic acid deficiency:* Warning— damage to internal organs may occur as a result of prolonged, severe folic acid deficiency. Additionally, extreme folic acid deficiency significantly increases the risk for certain types of cancer, notably cervical, colon, and lung cancer. Take 20 mg of folic acid daily. If you scored above 37, take 30 mg daily. Follow the aforementioned dietary advice. Consume absolutely no alcohol. Eliminate refined sugars, white rice, caffeine, and white flour from the diet. *Note:* Dosages of 5 mg and above require a prescription from your doctor.

Vitamin B-12

Death and despair were the stimulus for the discovery of vitamin B-12. Until the 1920s pernicious anemia, a relatively common disease of that era, was invariably fatal. Then came the dramatic announcement by Minot and Murphy that large amounts of liver, nearly one pound per day, cured the disease.

Researchers later discovered that liver contains not only large amounts of B-12, but it also stores a unique nutrient called *intrinsic factor*. It was actually this latter substance, which is an essential aid to B-12 absorption, that was responsible for the dramatic improvement of patients with pernicious anemia. By 1955 the most complex of all vitamins was synthesized.

Vitamin B-12 is also known as *cobalamin*. This name was coined after it was discovered that B-12 naturally contains the mineral cobalt. In fact, a cobalt deficiency in the soil may indirectly induce B-12 deficiency within animals.

Dietary vitamin B-12 is found exclusively in foods of animal origin, and the top sources are organ meats, muscle meats, poultry, fish, eggs, and milk products. Seaweed and fresh-water algae are the only known plant sources of this vitamin. However, evidence exists that absorption from seaweed and algae is less efficient than animal sources.

B-12 is required for the function of all nerve fibers, particularly the peripheral nerves. Thus, symptoms relative to the function of the brain, spinal cord, nerves, and muscles often dominate the clinical picture of B-12 deficiency.

Which of these apply to you?

1. dark circles under the eyes
2. chronic fatigue
3. swollen and/or inflamed tongue
4. chronic constipation
5. paranoia and/or psychotic behavior
6. memory loss
7. anemia due to enlarged (macrocytic) red blood cells
8. pale complexion
9. shortness of breath and/or difficulty breathing
10. lack of appetite
11. abdominal discomfort
12. weight loss
13. depression/anxiety
14. burning tongue
15. bursitis
16. bone spurs
17. nervousness, irritability, and/or agitation
18. loss of balance and/or staggering
19. numbness of the hands, legs, or feet

20. confusion
21. loss of taste
22. Have you had your stomach stapled, or has a portion of your stomach been removed?
23. Do you take antacids on a daily or weekly basis?
24. Do you take Tagamet or Zantac on a daily or weekly basis?
25. Do you avoid eating red meats?
26. Are you a vegetarian?
27. Do you regularly consume antibiotics (i.e. six or more dosages per month)?
28. Do you have a history of Crohn's disease, ulcerative colitis, or irritable bowel syndrome?
29. Have you been diagnosed with hypochlorhydria (low stomach acid)?
30. Do you regularly use cortisone or cortisone creams?
31. Have you been diagnosed as having low protein levels in your blood (low globulin, albumin, creatinine, BUN, etc.)?
32. Are you taking birth control pills?
33. Has part of your ileum (lower small intestine) been removed?
34. Do you feel like your feet are too big for your shoes when they really are not?
35. Do you feel like your legs are tight and don't move the way you want them to?
36. Are you over 65 years of age?
37. Do you suffer from premature graying of the hair?

Your Score _____

1 to 8 points *Mild vitamin B-12 deficiency:* Take a multiple vitamin-mineral tablet containing B-12 on a daily basis. Increase the consumption of foods rich in B-12, including

eggs, liver, lean red meats, and whole milk products. Eat liver at least twice per week. The liver must be derived from organically raised animals free of hormones, pesticides, and other toxic substances. Avoid pork liver.

9 to 18 points *Moderate vitamin B-12 deficiency:* Definitive evidence of B-12 deficiency is difficult to procure even by blood testing. However, blood tests are advisable with this score and should include hemoglobin, red blood cell count, MCH, MCV, MCHC, and a serum B-12 level. The latter test is useful only for individuals who take no B-12 supplements. Follow the previously mentioned advice, but consume the organic liver on a daily basis for at least one month. Then, eat it once or twice per week. Cook the liver no more than medium or medium rare, otherwise you will inactivate the most biologically active component, i.e. the intrinsic factor. Try also desiccated buffalo liver, six capsules three times daily.

19 to 29 points *Severe vitamin B-12 deficiency:* Warning—if left untreated, prolonged B-12 deficiency may result in permanent damage of the peripheral nerves. B-12 is required for the synthesis of the internal and external components of nerve fibers, including the fatty coating which surrounds the nerves (i.e. the myelin sheath). To correct this condition, follow the aforementioned advice. In addition, eat organic liver on a daily basis for at least two months and take eight capsules of desiccated buffalo liver three times daily. No alcohol can be consumed, since it destroys B-12 as well as decreases its absorption. Eliminate refined sugar from the diet. In extreme cases wherein the absorption of B-12 from foods is compromised, injections may be necessary.

30 and above *Extreme vitamin B-12 deficiency:* Warning—a deficiency producing these symptoms may result in permanent damage to the peripheral as well as spinal nerves. Aggressive

medical testing and treatment are probably necessary. See your doctor immediately and request testing for B-12 deficiency. Intramuscular shots of B-12 on a daily or weekly basis are required to rapidly correct this potentially serious condition. In addition, take sublingual or intranasal B-12 (1,000 mcg daily), since these forms are absorbed directly from the tissues into the bloodstream. Take eight capsules of buffalo liver four times daily. Oral forms are typically poorly absorbed by individuals with chronic B-12 deficiencies. Folic acid enhances the utilization of B-12. Therefore, folic acid supplementation is also warranted; take at least one milligram of folic acid daily.

Biotin

The essential nature of biotin was discovered by accident. In the 1930s researchers found that animals fed diets containing raw egg whites lost their fur in addition to suffering weight loss, paralysis, and, in some instances, death. The symptoms disappeared when the egg whites were cooked. Later, it was determined that these symptoms were due to biotin deficiency and that the raw egg whites contained a substance which destroyed the naturally occurring biotin in eggs as well as that stored within the tissues.

When biotin deficiency was induced, it created defects in three major areas: the dermatological (hair and skin), neuro-muscular (nerves and muscles), and immunological systems. Thus, biotin deficiency can result in significant health impairment. These ill results are due to the fact that biotin is a crucial component of several human enzyme systems. The biotin-dependent enzymes control such essential functions as protein synthesis, fatty acid synthesis/metabolism, white blood cell activity, and sugar metabolism. The fact that biotin is involved in the synthesis of fatty acids may explain why it is reported to be effective for hair loss, since hair consists largely of protein and essential fatty acids. Biotin is also heavily involved in carbohydrate metabolism.

Recently, researchers discovered that megadoses of biotin are effective in lowering excessively high blood sugar counts, as seen in diabetics. In some diabetics, biotin was so effective in normalizing blood sugar levels that the need for insulin was eliminated.

Like many other B-vitamins, biotin is synthesized by bowel bacteria. Antibiotics, which destroy bowel bacteria, may induce a biotin deficiency state. Good dietary sources of this nutrient include organ meats, egg yolks, legumes, and nuts. Vegetables, fruits, and grains contain little to no biotin.

Which of these apply to you?

 1. dandruff
 2. hair loss (from the scalp)
 3. cowlicks (tufts of hair which stand on end)
 4. alopecia (patchy hair loss of the scalp)
 5. mood swings
 6. lack of appetite
 7. intolerance to sweets
 8. nausea
 9. muscle pains/aches
10. weight loss
11. scales on the scalp and/or skin (seborrhea)
12. lassitude
13. depression
14. pallor of the skin and loss of skin pigment
15. delayed development (growth impairment)
16. dry and/or flaky skin
17. brittle hair or hair that breaks easily at the roots
18. lips which are constantly chapped
19. dermatitis (scaly)
20. poor muscle tone and/or muscular atrophy
21. muscular soreness

22. Do you drink alcoholic beverages on a daily or weekly basis?
23. Do you suffer from diabetes or high blood sugar?
24. Do you regularly take antibiotics?
25. Do you eat raw eggs regularly?
26. Do you have abnormally high cholesterol and/or triglyceride levels?
27. Do you consume refined sugar or foods containing biotin on a daily or weekly basis?
28. Do you have hardening of the arteries?
29. Do you have a current and/or family history of male pattern baldness?

Your Score ____

1 to 7 points *Mild biotin deficiency:* Increase the consumption of biotin-rich foods and take 1 mg of biotin daily. Avoid eating raw eggs.

8 to 15 points *Moderate biotin deficiency:* Take 3 mg of biotin every day. Increase the consumption of biotin-rich foods. Avoid raw eggs as well as refined sugar. Rice polishings are rich in biotin; consume 2 heaping tablespoons twice daily.

16 and above *Severe biotin deficiency:* At this level of deficiency an individual is vulnerable for the development of diseases/disorders associated with biotin deficit, notably hypoglycemia, diabetes, heart disease, male-pattern baldness, and dermatitis. Take 10 mg of biotin daily. If you are suffering from severe hair loss and/or diabetes, increase the dosage to 10 mg twice daily. Also, take 3 heaping tablespoons of rice polishings mixed in juice or water twice daily. Stay on this protocol for at least 90 days, and then reduce the dosage to 5 mg daily. Avoid raw eggs, alcohol and refined sugar. Add hefty portions of biotin-rich foods to the diet.

Vitamin C

If an individual could choose only one vitamin to take supplementally, it should be vitamin C. Unfortunately, in today's age it isn't easy to get the vitamin C we need by eating traditional food sources of this nutrient. Even so, many people believe that by eating a helping or two of fresh fruit every day, they are protecting themselves from becoming vitamin C deficient. This is not necessarily true. Furthermore, even though commercial orange juice is thought to be an excellent source of vitamin C, it may contain little or none. That's because cooking, pasteurization, and storage, as well as the addition of synthetic chemicals, destroy much of the vitamin C naturally found in citrus drinks.

Americans live in a world contaminated with a wide range of toxins, and these toxins, whether in the air, water, or food, all destroy vitamin C. What's more, the standard American diet is typically vitamin C deficient, and this is particularly true for those who consume significant amounts of deep fried food, sugar-infested food, and/or junk food. Since the majority of Americans follow such a diet, the fact that over 60% or more of Americans receive less than the RDA for this nutrient should come as no surprise.

Prolonged vitamin C deficiency may result in degenerative changes within a number of tissues, including the joints, spine, spleen, thymus, lymph glands, liver, adrenal glands, ovaries, heart, arteries, veins, testes, and thyroid gland. Vitamin C deficiency may occur within the white blood cells, and this leads to a significant reduction in their microbial killing power. A lack of it also causes a reduction in interferon synthesis, and this chemical is the body's most crucial anti-viral compound.

While scurvy is uncommon today, low-level vitamin C deficit affects millions of Americans. Those at highest risk for vitamin C deficiency include:

- patients taking anticoagulants
- patients who regularly consume cortisone
- patients in chronic pain who consume large amounts of pain killers
- cigarette smokers, their children, and their spouses
- chewing tobacco users
- alcoholics and drug addicts
- nursing home occupants
- individuals on long-term antibiotic therapy
- individuals taking aspirin on a daily or weekly basis

Certain individuals are at a high risk for developing vitamin C deficiency as a result of working around or with noxious compounds. A wide range of compounds destroys or inactivates vitamin C, whether these compounds come in contact with the skin, are ingested internally, or are inhaled (volatile compounds). A list of some of the workers exposed to vitamin C-destroying substances includes:

tanning salon employees
gas station attendants
beauticians
chemical and nuclear plant employees
nuclear waste disposal employees
paper mill workers
miners
truck drivers and heavy equipment operators
oil and gas refinery employees
employees of synthetic fiber and/or carpet plants
farmers who work closely with toxic compounds
dry cleaners

pressmen
water/sewage treatment plant employees
roofers and road asphalt/tar crews
plastic factory employees
carpet and/or tile installers
airline mechanics and ground crews
flight attendants and airline pilots
clerks in airports (due to toxic fumes liberated by jets)
rubber/tire manufacturing plant employees
battery plant employees
furniture refinishers

However, despite this extensive problem of toxic chemical exposure, vitamin C deficiency is common in the United States primarily for another reason: the food supply. Less than five percent of the daily caloric intake for Americans comes from fresh uncooked foods. As indicated previously, citrus fruits, unless eaten directly from the tree, are not necessarily vitamin C-rich. Most commercial grapefruits, oranges, and tangerines are picked green and ripened in large warehouses. Incredibly, the ripening agent is bromine gas, which is such a noxious chemical that if it is inhaled in sufficient amounts, it can maim or kill. In contrast, sunlight is a nontoxic ripening agent which dramatically increases the synthesis of vitamin C within the fruit. Thus, because citrus fruits are not tree-ripened, their vitamin C content is reduced significantly. In some instances these fruits contain no measurable amount of this nutrient. What little vitamin C they may originally possess is destroyed by the gas ripening process as well as by the various fumigants and pesticides that are applied to the fruit prior to shipment. Add to this vitamin losses during transport and storage plus the fact that fluorescent light destroys vitamin C, and it can be readily understood that it is possible to purchase citrus fruits devoid of vitamin C.

Gas ripening is so widely practiced by the commercial food/produce industry that only locally grown and/or organic produce can be relied upon as a guaranteed way to receive optimal amounts of dietary vitamin C, that is the amounts listed on food charts. Another option would be to pick your own wild berries and/or fruits or maintain your own fruit trees. However, that's impractical for the vast majority of Americans. Thus, vitamin C supplements must be utilized to fill the void.

To make matters worse, Americans are being routinely exposed to a wide range of vitamin C depleting substances. Anti-vitamin C agents inactivate or destroy the vitamin through a process known as *oxidation*. These oxidative agents include:

- coffee
- sulfites
- nitrates
- cortisone
- antibiotics
- aspirin
- Indocin, Motrin, Voltarin, or Clinoril
- radiation treatments
- antihistamines
- smoke from burning wood
- carbon monoxide
- chemotherapeutic agents
- glue vapors
- x-rays
- refined sugar
- radioactive dyes
- cleansers and degreasers
- black tea
- MSG
- food dyes (synthetic)
- birth control pills
- cigarette, pipe, and cigar smoke
- pesticides
- smoked foods
- chewing tobacco
- natural gas
- inorganic iron
- exhaust fumes
- paint vapors
- micro-waves

Negative Vitamin C Balance

As previously indicated millions of Americans receive less than the RDA of vitamin C in their diets. In addition, the dietary habits of Americans, as well as the environments they live in, expose them to a number of substances which destroy vitamin C. Yet, of all vitamin C antagonists cigarette smoke takes precedence; some 25 million Americans are heavy smokers. Cigarette smoke destroys vitamin C essentially at a more rapid rate than it can be consumed. The smoke from a single cigarette may consume as much as 40 mg of vitamin C. A pack wipes out approximately 700 mg: three packs, 2,000 mg. Virtually no one in this country consumes enough dietary vitamin C to neutralize that many cigarettes. Thus, smokers, even without considering any other vitamin C-destroying factors, suffer from an extremely dangerous condition: totally negative vitamin C status, a condition which leaves them vulnerable to a wide range of severe illnesses, including lung infections, systemic infections, liver disease, blood vessel fragility, heart disease, emphysema, connective tissue breakdown, and, of course, cancer. What's more, most smokers consume large amounts of coffee, refined sugar, and alcohol, all of which oxidize vitamin C.

Passive smokers fair little better. Those who are in the same room with cigarette smokers lose untold millions of molecules of vitamin C every time smokers light up.

Let's look at another example: the business executive who has a high stress job. Stress causes vitamin C to become rapidly consumed within the body and also leads to its loss into the urine. Without vitamin C the body fails to produce enough adrenalin, adrenal steroids, neurotransmitters, and similar substances which maintain normal cellular functions. The preliminary manifestation of this is fatigue. This forces the executive to pursue uppers; he/she uses sugar fixes, coffee, tea, cigarettes, alcohol, and even drugs in an attempt to achieve quick remedies for the tiredness. The morning begins with a cup of black coffee and a sweet roll: a zero vitamin C breakfast. The refined sugar in the sweet roll and the various chemicals in the coffee destroy whatever vitamin C exists in the body. Thus, the executive starts the day with a negative C balance, a nutritionally disastrous circumstance.

To make matters worse, the executive arrives at the job only to enter a smoke-filled room. Next, he/she attends a mid-morning conference, which happens to be a particularly stressful one. In addition to the cigarette smoke which permeates the air, there is a tray of doughnuts, cookies, and plenty of piping-hot coffee. He/she belts down another cup of coffee and half a doughnut. The vitamin C deficit deepens. Now the executive starts to develop the symptoms of a migraine but thinks it is stress-induced (it is probably due to sugar, coffee, or smoke allergy). Worrying that it might become severe and force him/her to leave work, the executive pops a couple of aspirin. What little vitamin C is left in the tissues is now thoroughly decimated. By noon the pain deepens; perhaps eating will make it feel better, he/she presumes. The executive orders a submarine sandwich with French fries and covers the sub and fries with ketchup. The sub contains salami, a nitrated meat. Nitrates aggressively oxidize vitamin C. Then he/she ingests another dose of aspirin and follows the sub with a cup of coffee. Immediately after lunch, sinus pressure develops; he/she swallows a couple of antihistamines, another drug which destroys vitamin C. To his/her surprise, the headache is worse, not better. What's more, the executive is now overwhelmed with severe fatigue and a sort of internal agitation. Migraine pain, fatigue, agitation, and stuffy sinuses all add up to prompt this person to leave work early. This is despite consuming six aspirin, which failed to curb the pain.

Even though the executive is now in the relaxing confines of home, he/she feels overwhelmed because of the stress at work and the stress of the sinus pressure and migraine. The executive was previously informed by a medical professional that alcohol helps digestion. Since his/her stomach is tied in knots, he/she drinks a couple of shots of bourbon before the evening meal. He/she continues to feel miserable, picks at supper, grabs a glass of milk, takes another antihistamine and three more aspirin, then retires for the night: sick, tired, miserable, in pain, stressed, and totally deficient in vitamin C.

Since the migraine will likely continue into the next day or for several additional days, these extreme dietary and drug habits will also be repeated. No one should be surprised if such an individual suddenly drops dead from a heart attack, suffers a stroke, develops a life-threatening bleeding ulcer, or is afflicted with some other severe disease. No one should be shocked if this type of person develops cancer at a young age. Just as vitamin C is destroyed by these dangerous habits, other crucial anti-stress and anti-cancer nutrients, which include vitamin A, beta carotene, vitamin E, B-vitamins, selenium, magnesium and calcium, are also depleted.

The extent of vitamin C deficiency in America can be illustrated by viewing some sample menus. The following pages list typical menus for American adults, teenagers, and children.

Adult's Menu   **Vitamin C Content**

Breakfast
Bacon and eggs
Commercial cereal sweetened with sugar
Skim milk
Glass of orange juice   20 mg

Lunch
Hot dog with bun, ketchup,
 mustard, and sweet relish
French fries
Fudgesickle   -0-

Snack
Can of pop (caffeinated)
Bag of potato chips   -0-

Dinner
Steak cooked well done
Instant mashed potatoes
White bread with butter
Salad made from iceberg lettuce and
 tomato wedges with French dressing
Apple pie ala mode
Cup of coffee with sugar added   7 mg

This is an example of a typical middle-class American family menu. The individuals of this "family" only received 27 mg of vitamin C, and this daily ration is less than the RDA. However, as with most American families, the diet contains significant amounts of refined sugars, food additives, caffeinated beverages, junk foods, and refined flours. All of these substances oxidize vitamin C. Individuals who follow this type of diet will develop a negative vitamin C balance, unless their diets are supplemented with several hundred milligrams of vitamin C each day and/or they consume large helpings of fresh, organically raised fruits with every meal. In this example there are no fresh fruits or vegetables in the menu. The final score is as follows:

a) Coffee: steals 5 mg
b) Sugar (20 tsp per day): steals 20 mg
c) Miscellaneous food additives: steal 10 mg
d) Inorganic iron (in flour products): steals 20 mg
e) Exhaust fumes (from driving to and from work): steal 20 mg

Total Negatives:	-75 mg
Total Positives:	27 mg
Grand Total:	-48 mg

The following is a menu typical for today's teenager:

Teenager's Menu	**Vitamin C Content**
Breakfast	
None	
(or)	
Can of pop and leftover piece of pizza	
(or)	
Bowl of sugar-sweetened cereal with skim milk	-0-
Snack	
Ho-Ho, Twinkie, or Suzi-Q	-0-
Lunch	
Hamburger with fries (ketchup and onions)	
Chocolate malt	-0-
Snack	
Apple	15 mg

Dinner
Roast beef (well done)
Baked potato with margarine
Canned corn
Orange juice drink (artificial flavors
 and colors; no real juice added)   25 mg

This teenager smokes (one-half pack per day), resulting in a loss of 450 mg of vitamin C. His/her diet is high in sugar, and this causes the oxidation of 50 mg. The white flour, with its inorganic iron content, causes a loss of 20 mg. Add to this the typical loss from environmental toxins and exhaust fumes and the total negatives are:

Total Negatives:	-540 mg
Total Positives:	+40 mg
Grand Total:	-500 mg

Now let's look at a typical menu for American children:

Child's Menu   **Vitamin C Content**

Breakfast
Cereal containing sugar
 (ascorbic acid added)
Skim milk
Glass of apple juice   7 mg

Snack
Cookie
Glass of milk   -0-

Lunch
Sloppy Joe with dill
 pickle slices
French fries
Kool-aid
Small orange   12 mg

Snack
Candy bar
Can of pop   -0-

Dinner
Spaghettios
Canned corn
Piece of baked chicken
Chocolate cake
Glass of milk   -0-

Incredibly, the total vitamin C intake for the child in this example is a pitiful 19 mg, which is barely one third of the RDA. To make matters worse, this child is consuming a number of substances which oxidize vitamin C, including sugar, inorganic iron, bleached flour, food dyes, artificial flavors, caffeine, MSG, and toxic oils (in the French fries). All told, these noxious agents destroy approximately 60 mg of vitamin C, fully wiping out the daily intake. In addition, the child's parents smoke freely both in the home and car. Add another -50 mg, and the negative vitamin C balance for this day becomes -91 mg.

Total Negatives:	-110 mg
Total Positives:	+19 mg
Grand Total:	-91 mg

In contrast, here is an example of a menu rich in vitamin C:

Menu	Vitamin C Content

Breakfast
2 poached eggs, lightly cooked
Bowl of oatmeal (not overdone) with
 raisins or black currants
Milk or cream
1/2 grapefruit
Mineral water   65 mg

Lunch
Fresh vegetable sticks (carrots,
 red peppers, zucchini and/or celery)
All-natural cheese dip
 (with non-irradiated spices added)
Poached salmon topped with
 lemon-butter sauce, capers,
 and pink peppercorns
Rose hip herbal tea   130 mg

Snack
Nectarine and glass of mineral water   10 mg

Dinner
Salad made of fresh dark greens,
 including romaine lettuce,
 spinach, green onions, and
 watercress (extra virgin olive oil
 and lemon juice dressing)
Roast beef done medium rare
Baked potato with butter
Steamed broccoli
Bowl of fresh fruits (strawberries,
 kiwi fruit, and blueberries)   180 mg

The only negative factor affecting vitamin C status in this example is the unavoidable inhalation of pollutants and exhaust fumes that occurs in a typical day.

Total Negatives:	-20 mg
Total Positives:	+385 mg
Grand Total:	+365 mg

Vitamin C is found in a wide range of foods but is readily destroyed by cooking. Top food sources include rose hips, citrus fruits, spices, bell peppers, broccoli, strawberries, guavas, Brussels sprouts, and dark green leafy vegetables.

Which of these apply to you?

1. easy bruising
2. bleeding and/or purple-appearing gums
3. lower back pain
4. arthritis or other joint pain
5. delayed wound healing
6. loose teeth
7. chronic fatigue
8. sensitive to extremes in temperature
9. thinning of the bones
10. nosebleeds
11. thinning and/or premature aging of the skin
12. liver spots
13. petechiae (tiny red blood spots in the skin)
14. heightened susceptibility to infections
15. hemorrhoids
16. insomnia
17. dryness of the mouth
18. dry, itching skin
19. swollen joints
20. loss of appetite
21. listlessness and/or apathy

22. depression
23. tendency to form plaque and/or tartar
24. Do you regularly consume aspirin?
25. Do you regularly take non-steroidal anti-inflammatory agents such as Motrin, Indocin, Clinoril, or Butazolidin?
26. Do you regularly consume birth control pills?
27. Do you take antibiotics on a daily or weekly basis?
28. Are you exposed to excessive quantities of chemical or exhaust fumes while on the job or during your travels?
29. Do you eat a limited quantity of fresh fruits and vegetables?
30. Do you currently use cocaine, crack, or heroin, or have you used such drugs for prolonged periods in the past?
31. Do you currently consume marijuana, or have you consumed it for prolonged periods in the past?
32. Are you a cigarette smoker?
33. Are you exposed to passive (second-hand) smoke on a regular basis?
34. Do you easily injure your joints, muscles, or tendons?
35. Do you take cortisone or apply cortisone cream on a daily or weekly basis?
36. Do you suffer from learning or reading impairment?
37. Do you have a history of hardening of the arteries?
38. Do you work in or near a nuclear facility/power plant, or are you exposed on a monthly basis to x-rays?
39. Do you see spots ("floaters") in your eyes?
40. Do you have a history of degenerative joint disease?
41. Do you suffer from growing pains (children/adolescents)?
42. Do you have deep pain in the bones and/or joints?

Your Score _____

1 to 7 points *Mild vitamin C deficiency:* The symptoms of vitamin C deficiency are often vague. However, to be on the safe side take 500 mg of vitamin C twice daily and increase the consumption of foods rich in vitamin C.

8 to 16 points *Moderate vitamin C deficiency:* Even with a moderate deficiency of vitamin C, collagen production is adversely affected. This leads to skin aging and cellulite production. Take 1,000 mg of vitamin C three times daily. Increase the intake of foods rich in vitamin C. Avoid refined sugar and reduce the intake of caffeine and alcohol. If you are a smoker, it is critical that you quit now in order to prevent further tissue damage.

17 to 26 points *Severe vitamin C deficiency:* At this level of deficiency a wide range of degenerative diseases may occur. These diseases include cancer, heart disease, arthritis, lupus, diabetes, and lung disease. Smokers must understand that if they don't stop their destructive habits now, they may ultimately develop cancer or heart disease. Or, they may be stricken with a severe debilitating lung disease such as emphysema. Follow the previously mentioned dietary advice and take 1,000 mg of vitamin C four times daily.

27 and above *Extreme vitamin C deficiency:* Warning—damage to critical internal organs is imminent unless the vitamin C deficiency is corrected. Take 2,000 mg of vitamin C four times daily. The frequent dosage is necessary to maintain consistently high blood levels. If the symptoms of vitamin C deficiency persist, increase the dosage to 3,000 mg four times daily. Consume large helpings of foods rich in vitamin C and strictly avoid all substances which destroy it. Be aware that at this dosage, innocuous side effects are possible, namely flatulence and loose stools. If you develop these symptoms, reduce the dosage until bowel function normalizes.

Vitamin A

Vitamin A is perhaps the most versatile and valuable of all nutrients. An entire book could be written about it, as it serves seemingly innumerable functions within human tissues.

Dietary vitamin A comes from both plant and animal sources. The type found in animals is vitamin A, while plants contain beta carotene, which is essentially two vitamin A molecules bound together by a chemical bond.

Animals cannot make vitamin A. They get it from eating plants. The beta carotene from plants, once absorbed, is split apart by enzymes within animal intestines to form vitamin A.

As many as 60% of Americans suffer from vitamin A deficiency, and if the deficiency becomes extreme, frank symptoms may occur. The widespread consumption of deep fried foods and various refined vegetable oils in the typical American diet is a major reason that the deficiency is so common. Refined oils destroy vitamin A both in the body and within the foods in which they are contained (see the Hydrogenated Oil and Deep Fried Oil quizzes).

To optimally utilize dietary Vitamin A, it is necessary to have an adequately functioning liver. The liver performs several crucial functions in respect to the digestion, absorption, and distribution of vitamin A, which are listed as follows:

a) It is the storage depot for both vitamin A and beta carotene. Over 90% of the body's vitamin A is found in the liver.

b) It is responsible for splitting stored beta carotene into vitamin A upon demand by the tissues.

c) It stimulates the production of bile, which is needed to unleash vitamin A, as well as other fat-soluble vitamins, from fatty foods.

76

d) It synthesizes the carrier protein, *retinol binding globulin*, without which the absorption of vitamin A becomes virtually impossible.

Vitamin A is essential for the maintenance of optimal immunity. Immune cells, as well as organs such as the thymus and spleen, degenerate in the event of vitamin A deficiency. The adrenal and thyroid glands are also highly sensitive to a decline in vitamin A levels; cellular death within these organs may occur if the deficiency becomes extreme.

Children are particularly vulnerable for developing immune disorders due to a lack of vitamin A, since their diets are often devoid of foods rich in vitamin A. Dr. Lendon Smith, a noted pediatrician and author, relates that children who seem to "catch everything that goes around" usually have significant vitamin A deficiencies.

Since vitamin A is found in two separate forms, it is widely distributed in foods. Top dietary sources include fish liver oils, liver, halibut, salmon, swordfish, crab, butter, cream, whole milk, whole milk cheeses, egg yolks, sweet potatoes, apricots, tomatoes, carrots, dark green leafy vegetables, peaches, dark cherries, red bell peppers, red hot peppers, cantaloupe, winter squash, and pumpkin.

Which of these apply to you?

1. weak or brittle nails
2. brittle hair
3. dry scaly skin
4. goose-bump like lesions on the back of the upper arms
5. acne, especially of the upper back and/or shoulders
6. lack of sense of smell
7. dry hair
8. increased susceptibility to infections
9. night blindness
10. growth impairment and/or short stature

11. thick, scaly patches of the skin and/or mucous membranes
12. poor coordination and/or loss of equilibrium
13. xerophthalmia (dry cornea syndrome; dry eyes)
14. dry mouth
15. slow growing hair and/or nails
16. inflammation of the eyes and/or sties
17. loss of taste
18. weight loss
19. loss of appetite
20. chronic diarrhea
21. conjunctivitis (inflammation and/or redness of the whites of the eyes)
22. Do you have poor fat assimilation/digestion, and/or do you avoid fatty foods?
23. Are you vulnerable to developing infections such as sore throats, ear aches, colds, or flu?
24. Do you consume one or more alcoholic beverages per day?
25. Are you exposed to excessive amounts of sunlight?
26. Do you consume deep fried foods on a daily or weekly basis?
27. Do you have or frequently develop open wounds that become infected such as varicose ulcers, diabetic ulcers, or bed sores?
28. Do you have a history of infertility?
29. Do you use castor or mineral oil as a laxative on a regular basis?
30. Are you currently taking cholesterol-lowering medications?
31. Are you taking prescription drugs which inactivate vitamin A, e.g. Coumadin, Synthroid, Motrin, Indocin, Voltarin, and phenobarbital?
32. Are you taking iron pills or multiple vitamins containing iron on a daily basis?
33. Do you take aspirin on a daily or weekly basis?

34. Do you have a history of nasal polyps?
35. Do you have diabetes?
36. Do you have a history of malabsorptive syndrome, colitis, or Crohn's disease?
37. Do you have a history of chronic pancreatic or liver disease?
38. Do you frequently develop corns and/or calluses?
39. Do you have a history of internal and/or skin cancer?
40. Do you have a history of diabetes?
41. Do you have hypothyroidism?
42. Are you currently taking birth control pills or have you taken them for five or more years in the past?
43. Are you unable to produce tears?
44. Do you have ulceration of the cornea?
45. Are your gums inflamed and/or sore?

Your Score _____

1 to 9 points *Mild vitamin A deficiency:* Vitamin A deficiency at any level must be regarded seriously. Treatment includes taking a multiple-vitamin tablet containing vitamin A (10,000 I.U.) plus an additional 10,000 I.U. of beta carotene. Be sure to increase the consumption of vitamin A-rich foods.

10 to 19 points *Moderate vitamin A deficiency:* In addition to increasing the consumption of vitamin A-rich foods, take 25,000 I.U. of vitamin A and 50,000 I.U. of beta carotene daily. Avoid refined sugar and alcohol. Eliminate refined vegetable oils and/or margarine. Extra virgin olive oil and/or unrefined rice bran oil are acceptable alternatives. Be sure to get your daily fix (or several fixes) of vitamin A and/or beta carotene-rich foods.

20 and above *Severe vitamin A deficiency:* A variety of serious ailments are associated with prolonged vitamin A deficit. These illnesses include immune deficiency, growth

retardation, osteoporosis, heart disease, atherosclerosis, emphysema, kidney disease, diabetes, prostate disorders, and arthritis. In addition, numerous eye diseases may be induced as a result of poor vitamin A nutriture. These diseases include corneal ulcers, conjunctivitis, night blindness, myopia, ulcerations, macular degeneration, and even blindness itself. In fact, long-standing vitamin A deficiency is the number one cause of blindness in the world.

To correct severe vitamin A deficiency, consume liver, the richest known source of vitamin A. Only organically raised animals should be used as a source of liver. Lamb's liver is the richest edible source and is usually less contaminated than beef or calves' liver. The liver should be cooked as gently as possible to avoid destruction of the vitamin A molecules. Eat it as often as you can, preferably every day for at least a month. In addition, take a multiple vitamin tablet containing at least 25,000 I.U. of vitamin A plus 50,000 I.U. of beta carotene daily. If you cannot eat liver or have no access to organically raised liver, take 50,000 I.U. of vitamin A, preferably from fish liver oils, each day for two months, then reduce the dosage to a maximum of 25,000 I.U. daily. If your score is greater than 26, take 75,000 I.U. of vitamin A daily for one or two months, and then reduce the dosage to 25,000 I.U. as a maintenance. Do not take large doses of vitamin A for prolonged periods. It is one of the few nutrients which can cause cumulative toxicity.[5]

---

5. **Warning**: Vitamin A supplements, including cod liver oil, must not be taken by women of childbearing age. The consumption of vitamin A supplements in megadose quantities during the first trimester of pregnancy has been associated with a variety of birth defects. If you are a woman with childbearing potential, only the standard quantity of vitamin A, as found in multiple vitamins (10,000 I.U. daily), can be deemed safe. However, vitamin A supplements are safe to consume after pregnancy is well established, that is 100 days after conception. A safer approach for women of childbearing years would be to consume natural sources of vitamin A such as organic liver and fatty fish (from unpolluted waters).

Vitamin D

The term "vitamin D" is a misnomer. That is because vitamin D is in reality a hormone, not a vitamin. The definition of a vitamin is "an essential nutrient that must be obtained from the diet." This definition fails to apply to "vitamin" D, since it can be synthesized in the human body, specifically in the skin. Known as the "sunshine vitamin," the D hormone, as it should be renamed, is synthesized as a consequence of the interaction of ultraviolet light with skin cells. When the light rays strike the skin, they provoke the synthesis of vitamin D from cholesterol, the latter being located in large quantities within the skin's oil glands. Once synthesized, the vitamin is absorbed into the blood or may remain within the skin. As little as one-half hour of sunshine per day may fulfill an individual's vitamin D needs. In contrast, deep dark tans may actually diminish vitamin D production, since excess sun exposure damages the skin cells which produce this nutrient.

Ideally, vitamin D should be included in the diet, even if the individual gets an adequate amount of sunlight. Top dietary sources include milk, egg yolks, cheese, sardines, mackerel, herring, salmon, tuna, halibut, and fish liver oils.

Unfortunately, over the last 30 years seemingly as much emphasis has been placed upon the potential toxicity of vitamin D as its benefits. As a result, the medical profession has neglected to emphasize the crucial role played by this substance in human nutrition. Only in the past decade have physicians and researchers begun to give it the credit it deserves. Recent research has revealed that vitamin D is of value in the treatment of psoriasis, eczema, osteoporosis, arthritis, hypertension, kidney disease, prostate disorders, and heart disease. While synthetic forms, such as those found in many food supplements and the type currently added to milk, may be toxic in high dosages, the natural forms are essentially nontoxic. One major reason for this is the fact that it is virtually impossible to achieve toxic dosages of vitamin D from eating food. There is an exception to this rule: cod liver oil. While the vitamin D in it is natural, one can overdose on it. However, the epidemic problem is vitamin D deficiency, not excess. In fact, recent research indicates that there is more reason to be concerned about the synthetic vitamin D added to milk products than the extra amounts individuals might be getting from cod liver oil or other natural vitamin D supplements. Even so, a teaspoonful of cod liver oil per day is a sufficient dosage for most adults.

There is another type of vitamin D of which to be wary: ergocalciferol. This synthetic version has the greatest toxicity of all types of vitamin D. It is produced in chemistry labs via the irradiation of cholesterol. Do not use supplements containing it. Look for cholecalciferol instead. The latter type is essentially the same as the one produced within the skin.

All of the vitamin D synthesized in the body is made from cholesterol. Therefore, diets low in cholesterol may cause and/or contribute to vitamin D deficiency. This brings into question the value of low cholesterol diets. Cholesterol is an essential nutrient without which a variety of normal physiological functions become impaired. In fact, Vitamin D is one of numerous essential compounds produced from cholesterol. These compounds include estrogen, progesterone, testosterone, aldosterone, vitamin K, and cortisone. In the case of a cholesterol restricted diet, deficiencies of all of these life-giving substances are bound to occur. Individuals placed on reduced cholesterol diets who are also taking cholesterol-lowering medications, such as Questran, Pravachol, or Lovistatin, are at the greatest risk for the development of cholesterol deficiency and, therefore, vitamin D deficiency. Tens of millions of Americans currently adhere to low cholesterol diets, and many of these individuals concurrently take cholesterol-lowering medications. All are at a high risk for diseases due to cholesterol deficiency, including cancer, diabetes, dementia, osteoporosis, lupus, adrenal insufficiency, immune deficiency, prostatitis, and even heart disease itself. One of the greatest ironies in "modern nutrition" is the fact that recent evidence indicates that a fanatical restriction of dietary cholesterol may actually increase the risk of heart disease, particularly in women. This is thought to be due to a severe reduction in the production of certain cholesterol dependent hormones, especially vitamin D, progesterone, and estrogen. Additionally, vegetarians and macrobiotic adherents frequently develop cholesterol and vitamin D deficiencies, since their diets usually omit or restrict meats, fish, milk products, and eggs, the primary natural sources of these nutrients. There are no vegetable sources of vitamin D.

Vitamin D is the missing link in the prevention of osteoporosis. It also helps prevent arthritis and may be useful in the treatment of this dreaded condition. Its role in these and other bone diseases is based upon the fact that vitamin D is the key nutrient for stimulating the absorption and metabolism of calcium. However, there is much more at stake as a consequence of vitamin D's control over calcium metabolism than maintaining strong bones. After all, it is calcium which stimulates the firing of the nerves. It is calcium which modulates the contraction of muscles, notably the heart muscle. It is calcium which maintains strong teeth. It is calcium which helps keep the blood clotting mechanism on schedule so that blood is neither too thick nor thin. It is calcium which helps control the growth of the cells.

In respect to its role in cellular growth there is mounting evidence that vitamin D helps prevent colon cancer. Researchers at the University of California discovered that people who consume vitamin D in their diets, in this instance by drinking milk, were 30% less likely to develop colon cancer compared to people with similar diets who drank no milk. The researchers emphasized the vitamin D content of milk as the likely reason for this lowered cancer risk.

Vitamin D's role in vision was recently discovered by New York ophthalmologist Arthur A. Knapp. He gave a group of patients the nutrient for several months. The result was that nearsightedness declined in over a third of his patients, and in many patients it was completely corrected. Dr. Knapp's conclusions were that deficiencies of both vitamin D and calcium potentiated visual decline as well as the formation of cataracts.

Vitamin D deficiency is common in the United States, and in certain high risk groups it is virtually guaranteed. These groups include invalids, mentally deranged individuals and/or inmates of mental institutions, nursing home patients, pregnant women, strict vegetarians, individuals with chronic kidney disease and/or dialysis patients, people living amidst heavy smog, and individuals who have been bedridden for prolonged periods. All of these groups have in common reduced vitamin D synthesis from a lack of exposure to sunlight and/or lowered dietary intake. Other high risk groups include allergic individuals who avoid eggs or milk products (milk products are a prime source of vitamin D) and individuals who rarely consume fatty fish. Additionally, the absorption and metabolism of vitamin D declines dramatically with age. Thus, it is usually advisable that individuals over 50 years of age take a daily dose of supplemental vitamin D, preferably from fish liver oil,[6] this especially being true for those who fail to get adequate sunlight. As little as one-half hour of sunlight daily may be sufficient to generate the minimum requirement for vitamin D. The best food sources of Vitamin D include yogurt, cheese, butter, liver, and fatty fish.

---

6. **Warning**: Be wary of consuming cod liver oil that has an excessively fishy odor; it may be rancid. If fresh, the smell will not be overpowering. Be sure to refrigerate the oil after opening. To prevent rancidity, add 400 I.U. of vitamin E to the bottle.

Which of these apply to you?

1. insomnia
2. irritability
3. rapid heartbeat and/or irregular heartbeat
4. nearsightedness
5. nosebleeds
6. chronic diarrhea
7. bone pain, especially in the legs
8. chronic upper or lower back pain
9. aching in the teeth
10. frequent fractures
11. cataracts
12. premature graying of the hair
13. scoliosis
14. muscular rigidity
15. muscle twitching
16. muscle cramps and/or spasms
17. convulsions and/or seizures
18. vague or migrating joint pain
19. easy bruising
20. soft teeth and/or tooth decay
21. thinning of the bones (osteoporosis)
22. chipping and/or cracking teeth
23. arthritis
24. delayed wound healing
25. bruxism (grinding of the teeth)
26. Do you have psoriasis and/or eczema?
27. Are you bedridden or were you bedridden for prolonged periods in the past?
28. Do you have fair skin?
29. Do you avoid eating fatty fish such as salmon, halibut, mackerel, sardines, and herring?
30. Are you a vegetarian?
31. Do you avoid milk products because of allergy or other reasons?

32. Do you have mitral valve prolapse and/or heart arrhythmia?
33. Do you have colon or prostate cancer?
34. Do you have high blood pressure?
35. Do you have acne, pityriasis, and/or rosacea?
36. Do you get little or no exposure to sunlight?
37. Do you have liver or pancreatic disease?
38. Do you take Dilantin or phenobarbital (epilepsy drugs) on a daily basis?
39. Do you live in an area where there is heavy air pollution?
40. Are you bowlegged?
41. Do you have an excessively high or low serum calcium level?
42. Do you have a low serum phosphorous level?
43. Do you adhere to a low-fat low-cholesterol diet?
44. Do you have a history of duodenal ulcer, or has your duodenum been removed?
45. Do you take Tagamet, Zantac and/or antacids on a regular basis?
46. Do you have celiac disease or gluten intolerance?
47. Do you suffer from muscular weakness?
48. Do you have difficulty walking or climbing stairs?
49. Do you have congestive heart failure or enlarged heart?
50. Do you have gallstones and/or have you had your gallbladder removed?
51. Do you have chronic kidney disease?
52. Do you have a cholesterol level below 155 mg/dl?
53. Have you been diagnosed with Osgood-Schlatter disease?
54. Do you have bone cancer?
54. Do you have a concave ("pigeon") breast?

Your Score ____

1 to 9 points *Mild vitamin D deficiency:* Eat foods rich in vitamin D on a daily basis and take a multiple vitamin containing vitamin D. Be sure to get sun exposure daily.

10 to 21 points *Moderate vitamin D deficiency:* Follow the previously mentioned advice and take an additional 400 I.U. of vitamin D daily. Eat a can of sardines or herring every day. Be sure to get regular sunlight exposure; at least one-half hour per day and no more than 4 hours per day would be ideal. Wear appropriate protective clothing; do not sunbathe for prolonged periods.

22 to 34 points *Severe vitamin D deficiency:* Consume hefty helpings of foods rich in vitamin D (fortified milk products, fatty fish, and eggs) and take 800 I.U. of vitamin D each day. Or, take one tablespoon of cod liver oil daily for one or two months, reducing this dosage to a teaspoonful daily. Eating fish rich in vitamin D is preferable to consuming cod liver oil, as the oil may become rancid with time. Be sure to get one-half hour or more of sunlight each day.

35 and above *Extreme vitamin D deficiency:* Warning—you are at risk for osteoporosis and may suffer spontaneous bone fractures. Softening of the skeleton already may be evident. Furthermore, a long-term vitamin D deficiency greatly increases the risk of cardiac disease, neuromuscular disorders, colon cancer, and bone cancer. Since fat malabsorption is the most common cause of extreme vitamin D deficiency, take the following supplements to improve fat absorption: Lipase 4 capsules (500 mg) with each meal; biotin 5-10 mg three times daily; Inositol 1 gm three times daily; granular lecithin 1 heaping tablespoon with meals. Eat foods rich in vitamin D on a daily basis. In addition, take 2,000 I.U. of vitamin D daily for at least two months, reducing the dosage to 1,000 I.U. as a maintenance dosage. Try to get a minimum of one hour of sunlight daily.

Vitamin E

Perhaps best known as the fertility vitamin, this nutrient is far more valuable than simply acting as a virilizing agent. Vitamin E is one of the body's most crucial antioxidants, acting to neutralize a variety of toxins before they can cause cellular damage. It is an invaluable aid for the prevention of a variety of diseases. In fact, research has determined that it may prove beneficial for even the chronic so-called incurable diseases such as arthritis, lupus, heart disease, Parkinson's disease, multiple sclerosis, and cancer.

Vitamin E is the key antioxidant for protecting cellular membranes. It readily dissolves into the fatty layer of cell membranes and, once there, acts to protect the membranes from potentially damaging compounds. This function illustrates the tremendous value of vitamin E in living organisms, since, once cell membranes are damaged, the cells usually die or become functionally incompetent.

The NASA astronaut fatigue syndrome is an excellent example of the cellular damage that can occur due to vitamin E deficiency. While in outer space, the astronauts are exposed to dangerously high amounts of radiation from the sun. They have no earthly atmosphere to protect them from the sun's potent ultraviolet rays. These rays pierce the astronauts' tissues like so many millions of microscopic sabers. Inevitably, the astronauts' cells absorb some of this ultraviolet radiation, and tissue damage occurs. The result is sick, tired astronauts.

The fatigue the astronauts experienced is somewhat like that seen in anemic patients. Researchers at NASA discovered that the astronauts were indeed anemic, and the cause was red blood cell membrane destruction by ultraviolet light. When the astronauts' diets were supplemented with vitamin E, this harmful reaction was halted, and the astronaut sickness syndrome disappeared.

Every year vitamin E is the subject of thousands of research articles. There seems to be no limit to the utility of this substance in the treatment and prevention of disease. Research has determined that vitamin E exerts the following functions:

- It protects the digestive tract against cancer-causing chemicals.
- It reverses the damage induced by toxic chemicals, such as carbon monoxide, sulfur dioxide, and petrochemical fumes, on the lungs and other tissues.
- It protects the skin from sunlight-induced damage.
- It helps prevent eye damage from aging, excessive sunlight, and toxic chemical exposure. Individuals who regularly take supplemental vitamin E are significantly less likely to develop cataracts than those who take no supplements.
- It prevents arterial and heart tissue damage due to aging or toxic chemical ingestion.
- It halts breast tissue damage from the ingestion of toxic fats (polyunsaturated fats; deep fried oils) and helps reverse fibrocystic breast disease.
- It blocks the growth of certain tumors (in the test tube), notably melanoma.
- It increases blood flow to the internal organs, prevents sludging of the blood, and enhances the heart's pumping ability.
- It increases virility by boosting sperm count and enhancing the fertilization process.
- It prevents cellular membrane damage from dietary toxins such as alcohol, cigarette smoke, and poly-unsaturated fats.
- It helps prevent bleeding disorders, such as placental hemorrhaging, menorrhagia (heavy menses), and nosebleeds, by normalizing blood clotting.

Vitamin E is chemically classified as a terpene. Terpenes are alcohol-like substances which readily dissolve in fat. That is why vitamin E is known as a fat-soluble antioxidant, and this is also why it is found primarily in fatty foods. A secondary source is dark green leafy vegetables. Top food sources include almonds, sunflower seeds, hazelnuts, avocados, cold-pressed nut/seed oils, salmon, and spinach.

Since vitamin E is found in significant amounts in relatively few foods, supplements are a convenient means of achieving optimal dosages. People living in industrialized countries need to take a minimum of 400 I.U. daily just to protect themselves from the ill effects of pollution. Individuals who are exposed to noxious chemicals in the work environment or heightened levels of toxins as a result of urban living should take larger doses: 800 to 1600 I.U. daily. One study determined that 800 I.U. was barely enough to neutralize the toxic effects of environmental pollutants and dietary polyunsaturates, which deplete tissue stores of vitamin E. Natural vitamin E is the finest supplemental source, and even though synthetic vitamin E offers the advantage of being less expensive, it is far less effective.[7]

Children are being exposed to higher levels of radiation than ever before in history. Most significant is medical exposure, for instance, asthmatics who undergo repeated chest x-rays. Of even greater consequence is a history of being x-rayed while still in the womb. Millions of women are x-rayed while they are knowingly pregnant or during the early stages of pregnancy before they are aware of the pregnancy.

---

7. Acceptable forms of natural source vitamin E include mixed tocopherol concentrate, alpha tocopherol, d-alpha tocopherol, vitamin E succinate and vitamin E acetate. For further information regarding the definition of quality vitamin E, refer to *Eat Right to Live Long*.

Other sources of childhood radiation exposure include:

- television and video games
- personal computers
- radioactive dials from toys and/or watches containing radium dyes
- medical x-rays
- radon contamination

Children's diets are notoriously low in vitamin E. White flour, white sugar, white rice, macaroni/spaghetti, pastries, candies, cookies, pop, and commercial cereals are all devoid of it. Since these "foods" constitute a significant percentage of the calories consumed by America's children, virtually all of them are severely deficient in vitamin E. Exposure for prolonged periods to televisions and video games, as well as to passive smoke from parents who smoke, only serves to deepen the deficiency. As a result, it is easy to comprehend why millions of children develop severe vitamin E deficiencies.

Nitrated meats, which are common foods on children's menus (for instance, ham, bacon, salami, and bologna are all loaded with nitrates), are significant vitamin E destroyers. Children usually prefer these meats to fresh meats and fish, such as organ meats, beef, lamb, or salmon, all of which contain significant amounts of vitamin E. The consumption of empty-nutrient foods, such as juices, pop, pastries, cookies, and candy, instead of fresh fruits and vegetables further potentiates the deficiency. What's more, the foods children typically eat are loaded with deep fried oils, margarine, and hydrogenated oils, all of which destroy this vitamin. Add to this the fact that inorganic iron, which is found in all white flour products, oxidizes vitamin E, and it becomes readily understood why nearly all non-supplemented American children are deficient in this nutrient.

Which of these apply to you?

1. cold hands and/or feet
2. tendency to form blood clots
3. easy bruising
4. swollen legs and/or ankles
5. varicose veins
6. leg and/or foot cramps
7. infertility
8. impotence
9. liver spots (brown spots on the skin)
10. muscular wasting
11. intolerance to dietary oils
12. cataracts and/or macular degeneration
13. Do you have liver disease?
14. Do you consume alcohol on a daily basis?
15. Do you consume foods containing white flour on a daily basis?
16. Do you consume deep fried foods on a daily or weekly basis?
17. Do you use margarine as a spread, or do you use margarine/shortening in cooking?
18. Do you cook with refined vegetable oils such as Crisco oil, Canola oil, sunflower oil, peanut oil, or "light" olive oil?
19. Are you chronically exposed to radioactivity (nuclear plant workers, x-ray technicians, computer programmers, policemen, etc.)?
20. Do you drink fluoridated and/or chlorinated water?
21. Are you taking cholesterol-lowering medications such as Mevacor, Pravachol, Lopid, or Questran?
22. Are you taking iron supplements or multiple vitamin-mineral tablets containing iron?
23. Do you eat white flour products on a daily basis?
24. Do you have a history of heart disease and/or angina?

25. Do you tear or injure your muscles or joints easily?
26. Do you consume snack foods, such as chips, pastries, candy bars, pretzels, popcorn, pop, cookies, etc., on a regular basis?
27. Do you have a history of chronic circulatory disease such as Raynaud's syndrome, vasculitis, atherosclerosis, or coronary arterial occlusion?
28. Do you have a history of Peyronie's disease (i.e. erection which fails to recede)?
29. Do you have hemolytic anemia and/or sickle cell anemia?
30. Have you had repeated miscarriages?
31. Do you have chronic obstructive lung disease, particularly emphysema?
34. Are you exposed to heavy air pollution?
35. Are you undergoing chemotherapy/radiation treatments?
36. Do you suffer from hot flashes?
37. Do you have fibrocystic breast disease?

Your Score _____

1 to 10 points *Mild vitamin E deficiency:* Take 400 I.U of vitamin E daily. Eat a handful of raw sunflower seeds every day. Increase the consumption of dark green leafy vegetables.

11 to 21 points *Moderate vitamin E deficiency:* Take 800 to 1,200 I.U. of vitamin E daily. Eat raw sunflower seeds or almonds on a daily basis, along with other foods rich in vitamin E.

22 and above *Severe vitamin E deficiency:* Warning—severe vitamin E deficiency increases the risks for a variety of illnesses, including heart disease, hardening of the arteries, lupus, Parkinson's disease, anemia, infertility, and immune deficiency. Take 1,600 to 2,000 I.U. of vitamin E on a daily basis. An example of a vitamin E rich snack would be two handfuls of raw sunflower seeds or hazelnuts daily. Eat a

large salad made with dark greens and topped with chopped raw almonds, hazelnuts, or sunflower seeds every day.

Vitamin K

Vitamin K is essential to our very survival. That is because there is a function dependent upon vitamin K without which life could not exist, not even for a second: blood clotting. Vitamin K controls this life or death function by stimulating the synthesis of blood-clotting factors in the liver.

Henrik Dam of Denmark discovered this nutrient and indirectly gave it its name, the initial "K" being derived from the Danish word "koagulation." His fascinating research documented how animals fed low-fat diets developed internal bleeding and thinning of the blood. In 1935 Dam provided final proof that Vitamin K, a component of fatty foods, is essential for the maintenance of normal blood clotting.

Severe vitamin K deficiency is potentially life-threatening, although such extreme reductions in vitamin K levels are relatively rare. However, that is only because the human body has a stop-gap; it can synthesize enough vitamin K on a daily basis to keep blood clotting normalized. Vitamin K is synthesized in the liver but is also produced by certain naturally occurring intestinal organisms. The intestinal organisms are of such major importance in the synthesis of vitamin K that a disruption in their integrity readily leads to a deficiency. According to Robbin's *Pathological Basis of Disease*, intestinal bacterial synthesis is "the most important source" of Vitamin K. Thus, drugs which alter or destroy the intestinal bacterial flora, such as antibiotics and cortisone, are a primary cause of vitamin K deficiency.

Recent research has delineated the importance of dietary intake for maintaining optimal vitamin K status. Top food sources include alfalfa meal, spinach, Brussels sprouts, cabbage, cauliflower, kale, liver, and lean meats.

Which of these apply to you?

1. easy bruising
2. bleeding gums
3. spontaneous hemorrhaging (bleeding from the ears, nose, or rectum, etc.)
4. petechiae (tiny blood spots on the skin)
5. bone loss and/or frequent fractures
6. poorly formed (sloppy) stools
7. intermittent and/or chronic diarrhea
8. Have you taken numerous dosages of antibiotics in the past?
9. Do you have a history of repeated miscarriages?
10. Do you avoid eating dark green leafy vegetables?
11. Have you had a portion of your small intestines or colon removed?
12. Do you consume chlorinated water?
13. Do you avoid eating red meats and/or organ meats?
14. Are you on a low cholesterol diet and/or are you taking cholesterol-lowering medications?
15. Do you have intestinal parasitic infection?
16. Do you have chronic candidiasis (i.e. chronic yeast infection)?
17. Are you on Coumadin or Heparin therapy?
18. Do you suffer from Crohn's disease, irritable bowel syndrome, dumping syndrome, or ulcerative colitis?
19. Do you take birth control pills on a regular basis, or have you in the past taken them over a prolonged time?
20. Are you currently taking antibiotics on a daily or weekly basis?
21. Do you have pancreatic and/or liver disease?
22. Do you consume alcoholic beverages on a daily basis?
23. Do you suffer from gallbladder attacks, or do you have gallstones?
24. Has your gallbladder been removed?
25. Do you suffer from gluten intolerance (celiac disease)?

26. Do your peripheral blood vessels burst easily?
27. Do you have a significant family history of stroke, or have you suffered a stroke?
28. Do you have spider or varicose veins?
29. Do you suffer from osteoporosis (thinning of the bones)?
30. Do you take mineral oil or castor oil on a regular basis?

Your Score ____

1 to 6 points *Mild vitamin K deficiency:* At this level correction should be readily achieved through dietary measures. Increase the intake of dark green leafy vegetables and take alfalfa leaf meal as a daily nutritional supplement.

7 to 15 points *Moderate vitamin K deficiency:* Take a multiple vitamin tablet containing vitamin K plus take alfalfa leaf powder on a daily basis. Consume hefty helpings of raw dark greens every day. Take an acidophilus supplement on a daily basis and avoid consumption of all antibiotics.

16 and above *Severe vitamin K deficiency:* If you are suffering from repeated episodes of bleeding, see your doctor immediately. Stop taking aspirin, cholesterol-lowering medicines, blood thinners, and antibiotics at once, since these drugs destroy vitamin K. Take a multiple vitamin containing vitamin K on a daily basis. In addition, take 1200 I.U. of vitamin E daily, since it helps conserve and regenerate vitamin K. Vitamin C and bioflavonoid supplements may also be beneficial, since they help keep arterial tissues strong and prevent bleeding. Most importantly, check with your health food store to see if natural vitamin K supplements are available. If so, take 2 or more capsules daily for at least 60 days. Consume friendly bacteria supplements daily with meals to reestablish bacterial flora in the gut. Avoid commercial meats, since they contain residues of antibiotics.

Calcium

Undoubtedly, calcium is the most well-known mineral and also the one most commonly taken as a supplement. Millions of women consume it with the hope of preventing bone loss. However, calcium has numerous additional uses as a nutritional supplement. It seems that every week this mineral makes the headlines regarding its importance in human nutrition. This is rightfully so, since every cell in the human body needs calcium to survive.

While too much calcium can be dangerous, all too often the problem is that people fail to get enough. Millions of Americans are suffering from the ill effects of calcium deficiency. The most vulnerable populations are adolescents and the elderly. However, deficiency in children is also common. A wide range of disorders may result, including attention deficit, growth retardation, tooth formation, leg cramps, nosebleed, and bone deformities.

Calcium is the most abundant mineral in the body, some 99% of it being found in the bones. Thus, the bones serve as the calcium reservoir. If there is too much calcium, the body deposits it in the bones. On the other hand, if individuals become deficient in calcium, the bones release it into the blood. This protective mechanism is necessary, because without calcium certain critical organ systems, such as the nervous system, heart, and arteries, would degenerate and death could result. Fortunately, calcium deficiency of this extreme occurs only rarely in the United States.

Since calcium deficiency occurs primarily at the expense of the skeleton, a number of symptoms specifically related to the bones and joints may result. However, because calcium also controls the function of the nerves, an endless list of musculoskeletal and neurological symptoms may develop as a result of mild to moderate calcium deficiency.

Severe calcium deficiency occurs most commonly in certain high risk groups. These groups include diabetics, cardiac patients, post-surgical patients, elderly individuals, Alzheimer's and Parkinson's patients, arthritis sufferers, and nursing home occupants. Additionally, certain substances antagonize calcium absorption and/or cause calcium loss into the urine or stool. These substances include:

aspirin	tetracycline
cortisone	calcium-channel blockers
chemotherapeutic agents	antacids

Cortisone is one of the chief calcium antagonizing drugs, since it causes massive mobilization of calcium from bone. With cortisone therapy, the calcium losses may be so severe that the entire skeleton becomes porous. In fact, the bones may become so weak that they split or crack spontaneously. In addition, people who fail to exercise regularly are at high risk for osteoporosis. Sleeping on a soft mattress also increases the risk.

Calcium absorption is dependent upon vitamin D. This vitamin can be consumed through the diet, but it is also synthesized in the skin, a reaction which requires sunlight. Thus, those who live in regions with short summers and/or people who rarely go outdoors are likely to be calcium deficient. Additionally, bedridden and wheelchair-bound patients usually develop rather severe calcium deficiencies. This category includes nursing home occupants as well as the thousands of bedfast individuals who occupy the hospitals. The risk factors for such individuals are extensive and are listed as follows:

a) They are usually taking drugs which impair calcium absorption.

b) They get little or no exercise and, thus, readily lose calcium from their bones.
c) They spend most of their time in bed.
d) They get little or no sunlight.
e) They usually receive less than the RDA for calcium and vitamin D in their diets.
f) Their diets are high in refined sugars, which disrupt calcium metabolism and cause bone loss.
g) They absorb calcium poorly even if taking it supplementally; this is largely due to the decreased production of stomach acid that invariably occurs in poorly nourished and/or elderly individuals; hydrochloric acid is essential for calcium digestion and assimilation.
h) They receive little or no food rich in vitamin A, a nutrient required for efficient calcium absorption and transport.

It is no surprise that spontaneous fractures of the hips and/or spine are a prime cause of morbidity and mortality in the elderly. There is a virtual epidemic of calcium and vitamin D deficiency in this population, one that cannot be corrected simply by drinking a glass or two of milk per day. These individuals require large doses of absorbable calcium and vitamin D on a daily basis.

Which of these apply to you?

1. joint pain
2. slow pulse rate
3. nervousness or irritability
4. tremors
5. twitching muscles and/or leg cramps
6. anxiety
7. chronic back and/or hip pain

8. vulnerability to fractures
9. loose teeth
10. tendency to form cavities
11. brittle nails
12. high blood pressure
13. numbness and/or tingling of the extremities
14. spastic stomach
15. muscular tension
16. chronic headaches
17. soft teeth
18. vertically ridged nails
19. Do you get little or no exposure to sunshine?
20. Do you have irritable bowel syndrome (colitis)?
21. Do you avoid eating fresh fish and/or milk products?
22. Do you drink three or more cups of coffee per day?
23. Are you a cigarette, pipe, or cigar smoker?
24. Do you regularly take cortisone or use cortisone creams?
25. Do you regularly consume antacids?
26. Do you regularly take tetracycline?
27. Are you on calcium channel blockers?
28. Have you undergone or are you currently undergoing chemotherapy?
29. Do you get little or no exercise?
30. Are you currently bedridden and/or wheelchair-bound?
31. Do you consume refined sugar on a daily basis?

Your Score ____

1 to 9 points *Mild calcium deficiency:* A mild calcium deficit is easily corrected by increasing the consumption of calcium-rich foods. Try the Calcium-Rich Vegetable Juice Cocktail listed in the recipe section. Eat foods rich in vitamin D for aiding calcium absorption. If you can tolerate milk products, eat two cups of yogurt or cottage cheese daily. In addition, be sure to exercise regularly, since physical activity aids in the deposition of calcium into bone. Supplementation may be

indicated; calcium has a calming effect upon the nervous system. Furthermore, it is protective against cancer of the colon.

10 to 19 points *Moderate calcium deficiency:* Follow all the recommendations for mild calcium deficiency. In addition, to further enhance absorption, take a multiple vitamin containing vitamin D and calcium along with an additional 500 mg of supplemental calcium. Walk one mile or more every day. For best absorption take supplemental calcium at bedtime, using calcium with vitamin C or lemon juice. Avoid substances which deplete tissue calcium: cigarette smoke, coffee, antacids, cortisone, soda pop, and refined sugars.

20 or above *Severe calcium deficiency:* This level of deficiency may not be entirely the result of dietary lack. Numerous disease processes may induce severe calcium deficit. Included are chronic kidney infections and other renal diseases, hyperparathyroidism, hyperthyroidism, hepatitis, cirrhosis of the liver, sluggish liver syndrome, and cancer. Notice the emphasis upon liver disorders; that is because this organ synthesizes calcium-binding proteins, without which this mineral cannot be absorbed. Additionally, vitamin D deficiency may cause calcium loss, even if the dietary intake of this mineral is adequate. To correct the calcium deficit, follow the aforementioned advice. In addition, take 1500 mg of absorbable calcium daily. Avoid oyster shell calcium. This type of supplement is poorly absorbed, and its consumption has been linked to kidney stone formation. Another form to avoid is bone meal, or ground bone, since it usually contains residues of heavy metals, particularly lead. Calcium citrate, hydroxyapatite, or calcium lactate would be preferable. Additionally, increase the intake of calcium-rich foods and drink the Calcium-Rich Vegetable Juice Cocktail daily (see recipe in Appendix B). Be sure to increase your fluid intake when taking large doses of calcium. Walk two or

more miles per day and/or be sure to partake in other exercises regularly in order to stimulate calcium deposition into bone.

Chromium

Chromium is perhaps best known as chrome, which is the metallic form of this mineral. Chrome obviously has no nutritional value. Yet, organic chromium, the type found in food, is absorbed and utilized by the body.

Chromium is essential for the function of the blood sugar regulating system. It aids in the absorption of sugar into the bloodstream and helps drive sugar in the form of glucose into the cells so it can be utilized as fuel. Additionally, chromium is involved in the digestion and metabolism of fats and proteins.

Chromium deficiency is common in the United States. This is largely a consequence of the refinement of foods, particularly grains, a process which results in the destruction of virtually all of the naturally occurring chromium. For instance, whole-grain wheat, rye, and barley are excellent sources of chromium, but when these grains are refined into flour, chromium losses may reach 95%.

Determining if an individual is chromium deficient through medical testing isn't easy. The deficiency simply must be presumed, since the American diet is devoid of it. A study by the U.S. Department of Agriculture found that the diets of 90% of Americans tested were deficient in chromium. This is certainly due to a lack of it in the diet but is also a result of the consumption of chromium-depleting agents, particularly refined sugars. An additional factor is stress, which causes a loss of chromium into urine and/or stool. Physical stress may wreak more havoc on chromium stores than even mental stress. The results of one study appearing in *Sports Medicine* (1987) showed that the urine of joggers completing a six mile run contained five times the normal amount of chromium.

Chromium is involved in the metabolism of fats and sugars. A lack of it results in the distorted function of insulin, the hormone that regulates blood sugar levels. In fact, chromium deficiency can ultimately lead to an insulin deficiency in addition to reducing insulin's effectiveness. The result is blood sugar disturbances, elevated blood fats, high blood sugar, and, ultimately, diabetes.

Chromium is found in relatively few foods. Fruits and vegetables contain virtually none, and most processed foods are devoid of it. Top sources include brewer's yeast, whole grains, rice polishings, eggs, and black pepper.

Which of these apply to you?

1. blood sugar disturbances
2. difficulty losing weight
3. chronic fatigue
4. intolerance to sugar or starch
5. tendency to rapidly gain weight after eating sugars and/or starches
6. cravings for sugars and/or starches
7. poor muscle tone and/or muscular weakness
8. chronic or morbid obesity
9. chronic depression and/or anxiety
10. craving for sweets, especially after meals
11. sudden loss of weight
12. episodes of shakiness
13. reversible tremors
14. Do you have a history of infertility and/or reduced sperm count?
15. Do you have high blood cholesterol levels?
16. Do you have high blood triglyceride levels?
17. Do you have elevated blood sugar and/or diabetes?

18. Do you consume refined sugar, as hidden sugar in foods or beverages, on a daily basis?
19. Do you regularly consume alcoholic beverages (4 or more drinks per week)?
20. Do you regularly consume white flour products such as white bread, buns, muffins, toast, pasta, crackers, or doughnuts?
21. On average, do you jog 2 or more miles every day?
22. Do you fall asleep after eating starchy or sugary foods?
23. Do you eat white rice on a regular basis?
24. Do you have a history of cataracts or macular degeneration?
25. Do you have a history of arterial blockage, hardening of the arteries, or coronary artery disease?
26. Are you nearsighted?
27. Do you have blurry vision?

Your Score ＿＿＿

1 to 6 points *Mild chromium deficiency:* Increase your consumption of chromium-rich foods, reduce your sugar and alcohol intake, and take 100 mcg of chromium, preferably as picolinate or GTF (i.e. glucose tolerance factor), twice daily.

7 to 13 points *Moderate chromium deficiency:* At this level tissue damage is likely to occur as a result of impaired sugar and/or fat metabolism. In particular, chromium deficiency has been associated with degeneration of the arteries. Obesity is also a probable result of a moderate deficiency. Take 200 mcg of chromium two or three times daily and reduce the intake of white sugar, flour, and rice. Avoid alcoholic beverages and sugar-sweetened drinks. Take 3 heaping table-spoons of rice polishings daily mixed in juice, water, or milk.

14 and above   *Severe chromium deficiency:* Warning—tissue damage is imminent if the chromium deficiency remains unresolved. Hypoglycemia, diabetes, morbid obesity, cataracts, depression/anxiety, cancer and/or heart disease all are likely to result. Eliminate dietary sources of refined sugar and curtail the intake of alcoholic beverages. Foods containing white flour or rice should be also eliminated from the diet. Take 250 mcg of chromium three or four times daily. In addition, consume 3 heaping tablespoons of rice polishings morning and night mixed in water, milk, or juice. Add rice polishings to the diet whenever possible as an additive to cereals and/or recipes. Try the Chromium Shake recipe in the recipe section of this book.

Copper

The first evidence for the essential nature of copper in human nutrition was discovered in 1928. A lack of it led to anemia in all subjects tested. Today, copper deficiency is relatively uncommon but only for one reason: copper pipes. Most Americans get their RDA of copper just by drinking tap water. However, not everyone drinks tap water, and not all tap water runs through copper pipes.

Deficiency of copper may occur as a result of a processed food diet. Additionally, certain groups are at an exceptionally high risk for copper deficiency. These groups include:

- those undergoing high-dose zinc therapy
- gastrectomy patients
- those taking multiple medications
- individuals consuming a high sugar diet
- cancer patients undergoing chemotherapy
- patients with chronic liver disease, including cirrhosis and hepatitis

- individuals with celiac sprue
- individuals who have had a portion of their intestines or stomach removed

Copper is an essential component of numerous human enzymes, including superoxide dismutase (SOD). Additionally, it works together with iron in the building of red blood cells. Thus, copper is an important anti-anemia factor. It is also involved in the maintenance of the health of arterial tissues, and if copper deficiency becomes extreme, degeneration of the arteries usually results.

For individuals with chronic arthritis, the "copper bracelet" may not be entirely an old wives' tale. This is because joint degeneration has been associated with trace mineral deficiencies, copper being one of them.

Perhaps the most common cause of extreme copper deficiency is the consumption of excessive amounts of refined sugar. In addition to being deficient in copper, sugar causes the loss of copper into the stool and urine. Another common cause of extreme copper deficiency is megadose zinc therapy. This is because zinc impedes the absorption of copper. Usually, dosages of 90 mg or more per day are required to artificially induce copper deficit. Anyone consuming large amounts of zinc should supplement their diet with copper. Top food sources of copper include rice bran, liver, red meats, whole grains, and mushrooms.

Which of these apply to you?

1. heart rhythm disturbances
2. alopecia (patchy hair loss)
3. skin rashes
4. diarrhea
5. fatigue
6. fragile or brittle bones
7. difficulty breathing

8. anemia
9. infertility
10. numbness or paresthesia
11. bitter taste in the mouth
12. poor wound healing
13. delayed healing of fractures or sprains
14. Are you a diabetic?
15. Do you have a significant family history of diabetes?
16. Do you suffer from hardening of the arteries?
17. Do you consume sugar, particularly fructose, regularly?
18. Do you have a high cholesterol level?
19. Do you have osteoarthritis?
20. Do you take 75 mg or more of zinc daily?
21. Do you perspire heavily?
22. Do you eat primarily processed foods?

Your Score _____

1 to 5 points *Mild copper deficiency:* Take a multiple-vitamin tablet containing copper and increase the consumption of foods rich in copper. Avoid all sources of refined sugar.

6 to 11 points *Moderate copper deficiency:* Take 4 mg of copper daily. Include large helpings of copper-rich foods in the diet. Avoid refined sugars and reduce consumption of alcohol.

12 and above *Severe copper deficiency:* Take 3 mg of copper twice daily. Eat copper rich foods on a daily basis; rice bran or polishings, liver, and soya products, are excellent sources. Curtail the consumption of refined sugars, particularly fructose, which is specific for inducing copper deficiency.

Iodine

It was nearly sixty years ago that iodine made global news as a miracle cure. Singlehandedly, it eliminated a disfiguring and potentially life-threatening disease: goiter. This is because iodine is an essential component of thyroid hormone.

The goiter belt of the United States includes primarily the states surrounding the Great Lakes: Wisconsin, Illinois, Michigan, Ohio, and Indiana. Prior to the introduction of iodized salt, goiter was endemic in these regions. Several Canadian provinces, particularly Ontario, Manitoba, and Quebec, are also a part of the goiter belt. All of these regions have one thing in common; they have little or no iodine in their soils. Thus, food grown in these regions was and still is devoid of iodine. For some people this may not pose a problem, that is if the individuals are consuming sufficient amounts of iodine in the form of iodized salt, sea salt, or foods naturally rich in iodine. Unfortunately, many people living in the goiter belt are placed on salt-restricted diets for health reasons. These patients are often under the care of dietitians, who painstakingly eliminate all traces of salt from their diets and, thus, artificially induce an iodine deficiency. Unless such individuals are consuming significant amounts of fish and/or seafood rich in iodine, a severe iodine deficiency usually results.

Patients placed on salt-restricted diets who fail to consume iodine-rich foods are highly vulnerable to the development of goiter and other iodine-deficiency diseases. Many of these individuals rarely eat seafood. Therefore, iodine deficiency is common and so are the diseases it induces: hypothyroidism (underactive thyroid), hyper-thyroidism (overactive thyroid), and goiter.

In some arenas the medical profession appears to have reverted to the Dark Ages, prescribing all manner of highly toxic substances for the treatment of disease. Radioactive iodine is a favorite noxious agent for the treatment of overactive thyroid. It is used to destroy thyroid cells. This method of treatment is based upon the belief that if the thyroid gland is overactive, it must be destroyed before it destroys the patient. Just why the thyroid gland is operating out of control is rarely investigated. No consideration is given to the fact that as early as the 1930s, hyperthyroidism was proven to result simply from nutritional deficiency, with a lack of iodine heading the list. Unfortunately, the ultimate result of contaminating the thyroid with radioactive iodine is to create a physician-induced and permanent case of under-active thyroid, forcing the patient to become dependent upon thyroid medication for life. Yet, the problem could have been quickly resolved if the iodine deficiency, as well as the other nutritional deficits which caused malfunction of the thyroid gland, would have been judiciously corrected. Thyroid-nourishing nutrients include:

potassium	pantothenic acid
tyrosine	niacin
magnesium	folic acid
vitamin C	coenzyme Q-10
thiamine	zinc
riboflavin	copper

What a crime it is that many a thyroid has been destroyed by radioactive iodine and/or other potent chemicals when a half pound of shrimp per day along with a few nutritional supplements would have entirely resolved the problem.

On the negative side iodine is perhaps the most allergenic of all minerals. Allergic reactions to iodine can be quite severe. Perhaps the most commonly occurring reaction is to radioactive iodine, which is the type used in electronic medical imaging as well as x-ray diagnosis and treatment. The iodine is utilized as a carrier medium for a radioactive tracer, which concentrates in the thyroid. With thyroid studies, a bolus of radioactive iodine is injected into the veins.

Some of this iodine is excreted via the urine. However, the thyroid gland aggressively concentrates the remaining radioactive iodine from the blood. In cases of goiter, thyroid nodules, hyperthyroidism, or other inflammatory thyroid diseases, medical specialists detect large concentrations of iodine in the x-rays. Other tests in which radioactive contrast media are used include cat scans, bone scans, and thallium heart scans.

Iodine allergies/reactions can also occur with the ingestion of dietary sources, including iodized salt, iodine-rich foods, and iodine supplements. A common reaction to iodine is acne outbreaks. However, reactions may be of a far more severe nature and may include asthmatic attacks, hives or other rashes, throat closure, shock, and even death.

Iodine's most celebrated function relates to its role in thyroid gland metabolism. Simply put, the synthesis of thyroid hormone is entirely dependent upon it, and this explains why nearly all of the body's iodine is concentrated in the thyroid gland.

When ingested, iodine exerts an antibiotic-like action. Studies have shown that white blood cells absorb iodine from the blood and use it to enhance their microbial killing capacities. This mineral serves an additional valuable function related to immune function: it prevents mucous buildup. It seems that iodine is necessary to keep the mucous that lines many of the internal organs fluid or thin. This is especially valuable for individuals suffering from lung diseases such as emphysema, chronic bronchitis, pneumonia, asthma, and/or cystic fibrosis.

Top food sources of iodine include sea salt, shrimp, crab, lobster, sea fish, seaweed, and cattle/fowl raised on iodine-rich feed.

Which of these apply to you?

1. cystic and/or sore ovaries
2. cystic breast disease
3. severe menstrual cramps
4. heavy menstrual bleeding
5. heightened susceptibility to infectious disease, especially bronchitis, pneumonia, ear infections, and/or strep throat
6. chronic fatigue or lethargy
7. morning fatigue improving as the day proceeds
8. chronic skin infections (boils, acne, fungal infections, etc.)
9. excess mucous and/or thick mucous in the throat
10. stuffy sinuses
11. cold extremities
12. muscular fatigue and/or cramps
13. stunted growth
14. coarse hair
15. reduced body temperature
16. mental sluggishness
17. Do you have an overactive or underactive thyroid?
18. Are you on a low sodium diet?
19. Do you avoid consuming fish or sea food?
20. Do you have a low libido (sluggish sex drive)?
21. Do you have a history of goiter?
22. Are you 20 or more pounds overweight and/or do you have a difficult time losing weight?
23. Are you a night owl?
24. Are you a total vegetarian?
25. Do you have a history of infertility and/or low sperm count?
26. Do you have cellulite?
27. Do you have high cholesterol, above 220?

Your Score _____

1 to 6 points *Mild iodine deficiency:* Increase the consumption of iodine-rich foods. Use sea salt in all recipes.

7 to 14 points *Moderate iodine deficiency:* Iodine deficiency impairs thyroid function and weakens immunity. Eat iodine-rich fish and seafood. Take kelp or iodine tablets as a source of iodine. Use sea salt with all meals and recipes.

15 and above *Severe iodine deficiency:* Crab, lobster, salmon, cod, mackerel, halibut, and shrimp should be regular items in your diet. However, try to purchase seafood from areas with less pollution such as Alaskan and Icelandic waters.[8] Add seaweed and/or kelp[9] to your salads and soups. Purchase iodine tablets or drops from your health food store and take two or three tablets daily. Use sea salt with all foods. Additionally, be sure to avoid the iodine antagonists. These substances, known medically as goitrogens, are found in certain foods, notably Brussels sprouts, soybeans, almonds, rapeseed, beans, peanuts, cabbage, spinach, turnips, carrots (and carrot juice), beets, broccoli, cauliflower, peaches, pears, flax, and kale. However, cooking inactivates the iodine antagonists and, thus, only the raw forms of these foods must be avoided. There is a word of caution. Certain individuals are highly sensitive to iodine. This sensitivity can result in potentially life-threatening allergic reactions. If you

---

8. Seafood from contaminated waters is a health risk for two reasons: contamination by chemicals, radioactive material, and human waste (sewage). Recently a rash of cases of food poisonings have occurred from consuming shellfish contaminated by such organisms as Salmonella, E.coli, and even cholera. If you consume seafood, rinse with large amounts of water, cook it thoroughly, and never eat it raw.

9. Recently, researchers have discovered that kelp from polluted waters is contaminated with heavy metals, particularly arsenic. In fact, certain individuals consuming kelp developed arsenic toxicity. Use kelp only if it is harvested from a region of low pollution.

develop any unusual symptoms after increasing your iodine intake, stop consuming the iodine immediately. In any case, if you rarely consume seafood and do not take supplemental iodine, be sure to introduce the iodine slowly. Despite these precautions, iodine is a natural substance and is well tolerated by the majority of individuals.

Iron

Iron is one of the few nutrients that is a two-edged sword; it can be life-threatening to have either too little or too much of it. Most people are aware of the primary result of too little iron—Geritol commercials took care of that. However, there is a paucity of literature concerning the dangers of iron excess. A little known fact is that iron toxicity is a major cause of poisoning in children (from overdosing on vitamin tablets containing iron). In addition, excess iron is a predisposing factor for a variety of degenerative diseases, including cancer, arthritis, heart disease, Alzheimer's disease, and liver disease. The excess iron accumulates within certain organs, causing cellular damage and even cell death. If cell death is extensive, organ failure can occur, which may result in fatality. Organs wherein iron readily accumulates include the bone marrow, spleen, liver, kidneys, lungs, brain, and heart.

In extreme cases of iron overload, the excess iron is deposited in every organ, in fact, in every cell of the body. This condition is known as *hemochromatosis*. A similar condition, *hemosiderosis*, is less severe but may proceed to hemochromatosis, the latter being usually fatal. If caught in the early stages, patients with hemosiderosis can be cured by a combination of several therapies. Most important is eliminating all sources of dietary and supplemental iron. Additionally, physicians often prescribe phlebotomy, or bloodletting, as a means of lowering iron stores. Iron chelat-

113

ing agents, that is compounds which bind and remove iron from the tissues, may also be prescribed.

Due to the dangers of iron overload, vitamins containing iron should be avoided, except by those who are diagnosed with iron deficiency. Pregnant, breast-feeding, and menstruating women may also need additional iron. Men should never take supplemental iron unless under a physician's care for iron deficiency diseases. Iron-free multiple vitamin-mineral tablets are now available at many health food stores. They may also be ordered by calling Nutritional Supplement Service (1-800-243-5242).

Iron is one of the largest minerals, molecularly. Thus, it may be difficult to absorb. The addition of acidic substances to the diet, such as tomato sauce, lemon juice, vinegar and citric acid, greatly enhances absorption. Additionally, vitamin C potentiates the absorption of iron. Top dietary sources of iron include organ meats, red meats, blackstrap molasses, oysters, almonds, cocoa powder, caviar, pistachios and dark green leafy vegetables.

Which of these apply to you?

1. chronic fatigue
2. lack of appetite
3. spoon shaped (scooped) nails
4. confusion
5. memory loss
6. lightheadedness or dizziness
7. rapid heartbeat after minimal exercise
8. inflamed and/or sore tongue
9. irritability
10. chronic headaches
11. fragile bones
12. difficulty swallowing
13. brittle hair and/or nails
14. depression

15. constipation
16. paleness of the skin, especially facial skin
17. sensitivity to cold
18. shortness of breath
19. tingling of the fingers or toes
20. sores on the inside of or around the mouth
21. vertical ridges on the fingernails
22. hair loss, especially in females
23. cravings for cold water and/or ice (chewing of ice)
24. Do you take antacids on a regular basis?
25. Do you drink three or more cups of black or green tea on a daily basis?
26. Do you have rheumatoid arthritis?
27. Are you anemic?
28. Have you suffered from heavy menstrual flow for a prolonged time span?
29. Do you take aspirin and/or non-steroidal anti-inflammatory drugs (i.e., Naprosyn, Indocin, Clinoril, etc.) on a daily basis?

Your Score _____

1 to 6 points *Marginal or no iron deficiency:* Many of the symptoms of iron deficiency are vague and, therefore, may be mimicked by other conditions. Always remember that iron deficiency is best confirmed by blood tests.

7 to 12 points *Mild iron deficiency:* Never take supplemental iron on the basis of a symptom quiz only. If you are concerned about being iron deficient, see your doctor and attempt confirmation through blood testing. Such tests should include a serum iron level, iron-binding protein, and a serum ferritin level. Ferritin is a storage form of iron and is an excellent indicator of the total body burden of this nutrient.

13 to 19 points *Moderate iron deficiency:* Blood testing to determine the extent of the deficiency is indicated. Take a multiple vitamin-mineral tablet containing iron (18 mg per day) and increase the consumption of iron-rich foods.

20 and above *Severe iron deficiency:* At this level of deficiency a measurable decline in red blood cell count as well as hemoglobin is likely. Again, blood testing is indicated. If anemia is confirmed (a hemoglobin of less than 13.0 in women and 14.0 in men), take 20 mg of iron as ferrous fumarate twice daily. Be sure to take 500 mg of vitamin C with the iron, since it greatly potentiates iron absorption. Additionally, take a multiple vitamin-mineral tablet, 4 mg of copper, and extra B-complex. Organic liver, particularly calves' liver, is an excellent source of natural iron.

Magnesium

Magnesium is one of the most underrated minerals in terms of its importance in human nutrition. It is an essential nutrient and is required for the maintenance of some of the most basic functions of life. Crucial organs, such as the heart, brain, and kidneys, are dependent upon it. A lack of magnesium is associated with a variety of diseases affecting these organs, including coronary artery disease, hardening of the arteries, high blood pressure, heart arrhythmia, kidney stones, kidney infections, pyelonephritis, depression, anxiety, Alzheimer's disease, and Parkinson's disease.

Traditionally, doctors have underestimated the role played by magnesium in the prevention and/or treatment of disease. However, sophisticated blood tests are now proving that magnesium deficiency occurs frequently in the chronically ill. The fact is deficiency of magnesium in America is so common that it should be considered epidemic.

Literally hundreds of symptoms, illnesses, and diseases may occur as a result of magnesium deficiency. In fact, a greater number of diseases have been correlated with magnesium deficiency than with the deficiency of any other mineral. This wide range of effects is explained by the fact that magnesium is an integral component of every cell in the body. It is second only to potassium as the most abundant intracellular nutrient. The immense value of magnesium in human nutrition is best illustrated by listing the breadth of its functions, which include:

- neurotransmission and neurotransmitter synthesis
- skeletal muscle contraction
- cellular energy production
- hormone and protein synthesis
- digestion of starches and sugars
- sugar and fat metabolism
- white blood cell synthesis and activity
- digestive enzyme synthesis
- arterial wall contraction/relaxation
- stomach acid production
- antibody synthesis
- bowel motility
- intracellular mineral transport

Magnesium is a large atom and, therefore, it may be difficult to assimilate. Furthermore, it is absorbed more readily from food sources than nutritional supplements. Additionally, certain disease states compromise magnesium absorption, including Crohn's disease, malabsorption syndrome, dumping syndrome, ulcerative colitis, irritable bowel syndrome, anorexia/bulimia, hypochlorhydria (low stomach acid), hypo-thyroidism (underactive thyroid), celiac disease, intestinal parasitism, and intestinal or stomach cancer. Drugs that deplete tissue levels of magnesium include diuretics, cardiac drugs, cortisone, aspirin, and antibiotics. Additionally, both coffee and alcohol aggressively pull magnesium out of the tissues. Top food sources include whole grains, red meats, fish and seafood, poultry, nuts, hot and/or tangy spices, and cocoa. People who ravenously crave chocolate may be magnesium deficient, since cocoa powder is one of the richest magnesium sources known. Unfortunately, chocolate is always combined with sugar, and sugar causes significant magnesium loss from the tissues.

Which of these apply to you?

1. heart rhythm disturbances (irregular heartbeat)
2. constipation and/or sluggish colon
3. chronic fatigue
4. muscles tear or injure easily
5. muscle cramps (or cramps in the bottom of the feet)
6. depression
7. muscular weakness
8. inability to control bladder
9. night sweats
10. excessive body odor
11. muscle twitching
12. lower or mid-back pain
13. muscular tension or tight muscles
14. dizziness
15. enlarged facial pores
16. uncontrollable sweating of the hands, feet, and/or armpits
17. painful menstrual cramps
18. PMS
19. restless leg syndrome (i.e. constant jerking or motion of the legs at night)
20. chronic knee and/or hip pain
21. cold hands and/or feet
23. lack of appetite
24. sudden episodes of loss of brain function (mesmerized)

25. nausea
26. rapid heartbeat (above 80 beats per minute)
27. carpal tunnel syndrome
28. nervous agitation
29. repeated tapping of the hands or feet
30. Are you easily disoriented and/or confused?
31. Do you have high blood pressure?
32. Do you have chronic diarrhea or sloppy stools?
33. Are you easily weakened by stress or are you physically intolerant of stress?
34. Do you have chronic arthritis?
35. Do you have heart disease and/or angina pectoris?
36. Do you suffer from headaches occurring prior to or during your menstrual cycle?
37. Do you have overactive or underactive thyroid function?
38. Do you have osteoporosis?
39. Do your bones fracture easily, or do they fail to heal after fracturing?
40. Do you suffer from epilepsy or convulsions?
41. Do you drink alcohol on a daily basis?
42. Do you have a history of kidney stones?
43. Do you suffer from chronic kidney disease?

Your Score _____

1 to 8 points *Mild magnesium deficiency:* Take 400 mg of magnesium daily. The recommended type is magnesium taurate, a specialized amino acid chelate which offers the best absorption. Avoid magnesium carbonate, oxide, and sulfate, because they are poorly absorbed. Increase the consumption of magnesium-rich foods, particularly dark green leafy vegetables, almonds, seeds, and hot/tangy spices.

9 to 16 points *Moderate magnesium deficiency:* Take 800 mg of magnesium daily. Restrict your consumption of refined sugar, white flour, white rice, caffeine, and alcohol.

Increase the consumption of magnesium-rich foods, adding them to every meal.

17 to 26 points *Severe magnesium deficiency:* A significant decline in tissue levels of magnesium increases the risks for a variety of diseases, including heart disease, arthritis, atherosclerosis, PMS, and high blood pressure. Take 1200 mg of magnesium daily in a dosage of 400 mg morning, noon, and night. If you are taking diuretics, see your doctor so he/she can wean you off them. Additionally, alcohol washes magnesium out of the body. Thus, consumption of all alcoholic beverages must be halted. Consume large helpings of magnesium-rich foods with every meal. Use magnesium-rich spices, such as cumin, basil, and cayenne, in all your cooking.

27 and above *Extreme magnesium deficiency:* Warning—this level of magnesium deficiency can result in cellular damage in a number of organ systems, including the nerves, bones/joints, heart muscle, brain, kidneys, thyroid glands, and adrenal glands. Because of the severity of the deficiency, magnesium injections may be necessary. Even so, it is advisable to take 400 mg of chelated magnesium 4 times daily. There is a word of caution. Magnesium can cause diarrhea. If you develop loose stools, reduce the dosage. Liberally add hot, tangy spices to your foods. Include in your diet Brazil nuts, almonds, cilantro, basil, fennel tea, sage tea, sesame seeds, peanut butter, figs, oatmeal, hazelnuts, and spinach.

SUPER-HIGH RISK MAGNESIUM DEFICIENCY TEST

This test evaluates the risks for diseases of a potentially life-threatening nature that may develop as a consequence of extreme magnesium deficiency. A reduced level of magnesium in the blood or within the cells has been associated with an increased risk for sudden death from heart attacks as well as strokes. Spasm of the coronary arteries, which can result in heart attack, has been proven in numerous scientific studies to be caused by magnesium deficiency. Recent studies document how intravenous infusions of magnesium can cut the death rate from heart attacks in hospitals by as much as fifty percent. In fact, its value in the treatment of life-threatening cardiovascular disease is so great that researchers are recommending that magnesium infusions be routinely given to all cardiac admissions. The magnesium level within the coronary arteries and/or heart muscle cells is usually severely depressed in heart-attack patients. Thus, magnesium infusions should be available in all ambulances, emergency rooms, and coronary units. There is good reason for this prescription: If the magnesium infusions were given, the need for high-risk invasive procedures, such as cardiac catheterization, coronary angioplasty, and bypass surgery, would be greatly curtailed. Magnesium-deficient individuals also suffer from a heightened incidence of stroke, high blood pressure, dementia, multiple sclerosis, anxiety/depression, Parkinson's disease, and arthritis.

Which of these apply to you?

1. Do you exclusively drink reverse osmosis, softened, or distilled water (two or more glasses per day)?
2. Do you drink four or more cups of coffee daily?
3. Do you drink four or more cups of hot tea or iced tea daily?
4. Do you consume sweets often?
5. Do you eat refined sugar hidden in foods? (See pages 207-216 for a comprehensive listing of such foods.)
6. Do you eat white flour and white rice products, while avoiding whole grains?
7. Do you drink one or more alcoholic beverages daily?

8. Do you smoke 1/2 pack or more of cigarettes per day?
9. Do you use chewing tobacco?
10. Do you drink 2 or more cans of pop per day?
11. Do you take diuretics on a daily or weekly basis?
12. Do you take aspirin on a daily or weekly basis?
13. Do you take Tagamet or Zantac on a daily or weekly basis?
14. Do you use antacids on a daily basis?
15. Do you regularly use laxatives?
16. Do you take tetracycline on a daily or weekly basis?
17. Do you have a family history of heart disease and/or have you been diagnosed with coronary artery/heart disease?
18. Do you have high blood pressure (above 140/90)?
19. Do you suffer from chronic diarrhea, Crohn's disease, and/or ulcerative colitis?
20. Do you have restless leg syndrome and/or night-time leg cramps?
21. Do you snore excessively, and/or do you experience sleep apnea?
22. Do you suffer from angina attacks?
23. Do you take one or more heart medicines besides diuretics on a daily basis?
24. Do you have a history of muscle tearing?
25. Do you work with heavy metals, i.e. cadmium, mercury, lead, etc.?
26. Do you have severe leg, foot, and/or toe cramps?
27. Have you had one or more heart attacks in the past decade?
28. Do you have overactive or underactive thyroid function?
29. Do you have kidney stones, or have you had them in the past?

Your Score ____

Any score above five indicates you are at a high risk for developing severe magnesium deficiency. Individuals who score above ten are at an extremely high risk, and if such individuals have a family history of heart disease, it is critical to make lifestyle alterations immediately. Follow the same instructions as were listed for the previous magnesium quiz. A score above 18 is of great concern; the risk for sudden death from cardiac disease is astronomically high. Individuals who score above ten should see a physician and have blood tests for determining magnesium levels. Magnesium is an intracellular nutrient. Therefore, the serum level generally provides an inaccurate picture of tissue stores. Thus, both serum and intracellular levels should be assayed. However, blood tests are not the complete answer. It is possible to develop significant magnesium deficiency even though blood tests are normal. Thus, the clinical picture, that is the symptoms and patient history, must be used as the final determinant for assessing the need for magnesium supplementation.

Manganese

Manganese is one of the least studied and understood of all nutrients. Nonetheless, its role in human nutrition is highly significant, as demonstrated by the crippling disease, a form of joint degeneration, that results from experimentally induced manganese deficiency. As with other trace elements, manganese's primary role is that it is an enzyme activator. Dozens of enzymes, each with its own unique function, are dependent upon manganese for optimal activity. For instance, the enzymes involved in cholesterol synthesis are manganese dependent, as are those involved in the synthesis of cartilage and bone. Regarding the latter, the mucopolysaccharides, substances necessary for the formation of strong connective tissues, cannot be produced in the event of manganese deficiency.

Perhaps the most thoroughly documented and characteristic result of mild manganese deficiency is a specific syndrome of the joints known as *slipped tendon disease* or *perosis*. This is the result of a lack of skeletal maturation, leading to a slipping of the tendons off the joint and causing the characteristic "clicking" noise. These abnormalities are usually reversed by supplementing the diet with chelated manganese and manganese-rich foods.

Manganese is poorly absorbed from dietary sources. As much as 98% of ingested manganese is lost in the feces. Supplemental sources often fail to correct this, although chelated manganese products offer the best potential for absorption.

Which of these apply to you?

1. creaking and/or clicking of the joints
2. bone pain
3. arthritis and/or joint pain
4. infertility
5. thinning of the bones
6. brittle bones
7. increased susceptibility to infections
8. chronic knee, hip, and/or ankle pain
9. joints which are easily injured
10. Are you a vegetarian?
11. Do you consume large amounts of bran, particularly wheat bran?
12. Do you have short stature (height under 5 feet) and/or growth impairment?
13. Are you a diabetic, and/or have you been diagnosed with an elevated blood sugar level?
14. Have you been diagnosed with hypoglycemia by blood testing (abnormal glucose tolerance test)?

15. Do you have a history of hepatitis and/or cirrhosis of the liver?
16. Do you consume sugar, pop, or candy on a daily or weekly basis?
17. Do you have low or high cholesterol?
18. Do you have a tendency to frequently sprain or injure your joints?
19. Do you have gout?
20. Are you obese?
21. Do you have a fracture or severe structural injury which has failed to heal?
22. Do you suffer from a blood-clotting abnormality?
23. Have you had a portion of your small intestine removed?
24. Do you have low levels of blood proteins, i.e. reduced globulin or albumin?

Your Score _____

1 to 4 points *Mild manganese deficiency:* Take 2 mg of chelated manganese and/or a multiple-vitamin/mineral containing manganese on a daily basis.

5 to 12 points *Moderate manganese deficiency:* Take 3 mg of chelated manganese morning and night and increase the consumption of manganese-rich foods. Avoid consuming the brans of grains; they contain phytates, which bind to manganese and prevent its absorption. Take 3 heaping tablespoons of rice polishings daily.

13 and above *Severe manganese deficiency:* Take 3 mg of manganese three times daily (a total of 9 mg). To help enhance absorption, take 2 tablespoons of lemon juice with each dosage. Increase the consumption of manganese-rich foods such as legumes, fresh meats, spices, blueberries, ginger, brown rice, and nuts. Avoid dietary sources of phytates (e.g. whole wheat, corn bran, and oat bran). Drink

mineral water and avoid mineral depleted water, i.e. reverse osmosis, distilled, and soft water. Take 4 heaping table-spoons of rice polishings twice daily.

Phosphorus

Phosphorus is a sort of Dr. Jekyll and Mr. Hyde of the minerals. This is because it is required for survival, yet can deal death. For instance, the flame in incandescent bulbs is white phosphorus, the heart of a match is made from red phosphorus, and certain pesticides are made from organic phosphate. However, without phosphorus, cells fail to divide, hearts stop beating, and reproduction halts.

Comprising approximately 1% of body weight, phosphorus is one of the most abundant substances in the human body. In fact, by itself it accounts for nearly one-fourth of the body's total mineral content. Of this amount 80% is bound to the bones and is a component of teeth.

Phosphorus is closely related to calcium in human nutrition. Like calcium, it requires vitamin D for absorption. A deficiency or an excess of phosphorus can upset calcium balance. Normally, the proportion of calcium to phosphorus in the bone is 2:1. However, the ratio within the soft tissues is 1 molecule of calcium for every 20 molecules of phosphorus.

Dietary intake can play a major role in affecting tissue concentration of phosphate. Yet, few nutritional manuals emphasize the dietary need for phosphorus. Ensminger, et al., authors of *Food and Nutrition Encyclopedia*, aptly describe the crucial nature of phosphorus within the human body by stating: "Among the minerals essential to life, *none plays a more central role*...It is found...in every cell; and *it is involved in almost all, if not all, metabolic reactions* (italics mine)." Ensminger lists the functions of phosphorus as follows:

126

- It is required for bone formation and regeneration
- It is important in the development of teeth
- It is essential for normal milk secretion
- It is important for building muscle tissue
- It is involved in the synthesis of the genetic materials (RNA & DNA)
- It helps maintain acid-base and osmotic balance in the blood and within the cells
- It is essential for amino acid/protein metabolism
- It aids in the transport of fatty acids within the tissues
- It is crucial for the production of energy within the cells and muscles, including the heart
- It is an activator of many human enzyme systems

The proper utilization/absorption of phosphorus is dependent upon several factors. Phosphorous should ideally be consumed in foods, like milk products, in a 2:1 ratio of calcium to phosphorous. It should also be present in a bio-available form. For instance, the phosphorus found in milk products and eggs is highly absorbable, while that found in whole grains is poorly absorbed. The latter contain fibrous compounds called phytates, which bind phosphates irreversibly. Thirdly, sufficient vitamin D must be available to ensure adequate calcium and phosphorus absorption from the gut. In fact, when sufficient vitamin D is available, the ratio of calcium to phosphorus becomes less crucial.

Phosphorus is found in a wide range of foods. Top sources include cheese, wheat germ, peanut flour, pumpkin and squash seeds, rice bran, rice polishings, soybean flour, organic liver, almonds, pistachios, and sunflower seeds.

Which of these apply to you?

1. lack of appetite
2. anxiety
3. bone pain

4. loose teeth
5. teeth which crack and/or chip
6. irritability
7. numbness of the extremities
8. tremors
9. extreme fatigue
10. muscular weakness
11. swollen joints
12. chronic toothaches
13. gum disease (pyorrhea)
14. sluggish mental function
15. Do you consume refined sugar on a daily basis?
16. Do you avoid eating fresh vegetables, nuts, and seeds?
17. Do you have a history of infertility or low sperm count?
18. Do you have a history of coronary artery and/or heart disease?
19. Do you have osteoporosis?
20. Do you have more than four cavities?
21. Do you suffer from chronic joint pain (arthritis)?
22. Do you take antacids on a regular basis?
23. Do you have a duodenal ulcer, or have you had your duodenum removed?
24. Do you take cortisone orally on a regular basis?
25. Do you take iron pills on a daily basis?
26. Do you have chronic kidney problems?
27. Is your serum calcium low?
28. Do you have a history of a slipped or ruptured disk?
29. Do you follow a vegetarian diet devoid of milk products?
30. Do you have a problem building muscle tissue?
31. Have you experienced pica (desire to eat soil, clay, hair, etc.)?

Your Score ____

1 to 5 points *Mild Phosphorus deficiency:* A lack of phosphorus impairs energy production within every cell and

organ of the body. The phosphorus deficiency can usually be corrected by increasing the intake of foods rich in this nutrient such as whole grains, almonds, pumpkin seeds, squash seeds, rice polishings, filberts, egg yolks, lean meats, and fresh fish.

6 to 12 points *Moderate phosphorus deficiency:* In addition to the aforementioned take a multiple vitamin-mineral tablet containing phosphorus as well as vitamin D. Increase the consumption of vitamin D-rich foods, since this nutrient controls the rate at which phosphorus is absorbed. Eat snacks rich in phosphorus such as pumpkin seeds, sunflower seeds, pistachios, rice bran cookies, and cheese.

13 and above *Severe phosphorus deficiency:* Severe phosphorus deficiency may be a clue to the existence of hormonal disturbances. The parathyroid gland, which is located behind the thyroid gland at the back of the throat, produces parathyroid hormone. This hormone exerts potent control over the metabolism as well as absorption of phosphorus. Thus, a deficiency of this hormone leads to a decline in blood phosphorus levels. The adrenal glands also modulate phosphorus metabolism. Thus, a persistently low blood phosphorus level, despite attempts at dietary correction, is a signal of the existence of significant hormonal insufficiencies.

To correct this deficiency follow the previously mentioned advice and take 1,000 mg of phosphorus each day. In addition, take 800 to 1200 I.U. of vitamin D on a daily basis. Prolonged consumption of antacids induces phosphorus depletion which may be so severe that it is life-threatening. This syndrome is characterized by weakness, loss of appetite, and bone pain. Avoid antacids, cortisone, alcohol, refined sugar, and iron supplements, all of which impede phosphorus absorption. It may be necessary to monitor phosphorus status via blood testing. If the phosphorus level fails to normalize, medical evaluation for hormonal deficiencies may be necessary.

Potassium

No mineral can be deemed more crucial for survival than potassium. Without it, death rapidly results from sudden cardiac arrest. Potassium is the heart's nerve firing agent, initiating impulses to stimulate contraction of the heart muscle fibers. Therefore, the heart is dependent upon this mineral in order to pump in its unending fashion. Moreover, potassium helps control the function of every nerve in the body. Thus, a deficiency of this mineral would have a negative impact upon the function of every organ, in fact, every cell in the body.

Fresh tree-ripened fruits and vegetables are rich in potassium, but the top sources on a per weight basis are spices, particularly coriander, cumin, basil, parsley, ginger, hot pepper, dill weed, tarragon, paprika, and turmeric. Nuts, seeds, and legumes are also rich sources.

Potassium deficiency is a proven contributing cause of a number of illnesses, including:

arthritis	irritable bowel syndrome
kidney stones	Alzheimer's disease
atrial fibrillation	multiple sclerosis
celiac disease	myasthenia gravis
bundle branch block	Crohn's disease
high blood pressure	lupus
coronary artery disease	atherosclerosis
ulcerative colitis	diabetes
hypothyroidism	stroke
adrenal insufficiency	

Individuals who are taking high blood pressure medications are most vulnerable to developing potassium deficiency, since these agents cause the spillage of large quantities of potassium into the urine. Physicians often attempt to minimize this by prescribing potassium-sparing diuretics. However, the most commonly prescribed diuretics aggressively deplete tissue stores of potassium, causing a drug-induced systemic potassium deficiency. The thiazide diuretics, a category which includes Diazide and chlorothiazide, cause the loss of untold millions of molecules of potassium for every pill taken. This is one reason that diuretic usage is associated with sudden death syndrome. The fact is certain studies, including the MRFIT trial reported in the journal *Science* (October 1982), warn of the dangers of long-term diuretic usage. Such studies document how individuals who take diuretics for moderately high blood pressure live significantly longer than hypertensive patients who take medications.

Which of these apply to you?

1. acne
2. arthritis and/or swollen joints
3. constipation
4. impaired intellect
5. depression
6. memory loss
7. edema (swelling) of the extremities
8. agitation and/or irritability
9. low blood pressure
10. irregular heartbeat
11. rapid heartbeat
12. frequent urination with large volumes
13. blood sugar disturbances
14. constant fatigue
15. muscular weakness
16. nervousness
17. muscle cramps
18. lightheadedness and/or episodes of fainting
19. twitching of the muscles and/or tremors
20. intolerance to exercise and/or lack of a desire to exercise
21. poor appetite

22. chronic headaches
23. sudden episodes of paralysis
24. Do you consume alcohol on a daily basis?
25. Do you consume fresh fruits, vegetables, nuts, and seeds only occasionally?
26. Do you take antacids or Zantac/Tagamet on a daily basis?
27. Do you use diuretics on a daily or weekly basis?
28. Do you have high blood pressure (greater than 140/90)?
29. Have you had a stroke, or do you suffer from TIAs (transient ischemic attacks)?
30. Do you have a history of angina, heart disease, and/or hardening of the arteries?
31. Do you consume aspirin, Motrin, or similar anti-inflammatory drugs on a daily or weekly basis?
32. Do you take commercial laxatives daily or weekly?
33. Do you suffer from chronic or intermittent diarrhea?
34. Are you currently taking drugs containing cortisone?
35. Do you consume refined sugars on a daily basis?
36. Do you experience abdominal bloating?
37. Do you have swelling of the eyelids or swelling under the eyes?
38. Do you vomit frequently (once a week or more)?
39. Are you a diabetic?

Your Score _____

1 to 9 points *Mild potassium deficiency:* Enrich the diet with top food sources of potassium. In addition, take a multiple-mineral tablet containing potassium. Try the Potassium Shake recipes in the recipe section.

10 to 21 points *Moderate potassium deficiency:* In addition to the previously mentioned advice, take a daily dosage of 1 or 2 tablets of potassium gluconate twice daily.

22 and above *Severe potassium deficiency:* Warning—severe potassium deficit may lead to cardiac rhythm disturbances. If the blood potassium level drops excessively low, sudden cardiac standstill may result. Before beginning supplementation you should have your blood potassium level assessed. If blood levels are normal or slightly depressed, take 2 or 3 potassium gluconate tablets twice daily. In the event of severe potassium deficiency medical intervention is necessary. Proper care might include potassium medication plus frequent monitoring of the blood potassium level. However, there is a word of caution: potassium drugs, especially tablets, may be caustic and can cause ulcerations of the intestines. To avoid this, opt for liquid forms of potassium or utilize less toxic forms such as the non-prescription potassium gluconate. Eat potassium-rich foods every day. Prepare large batches of the potassium-rich fruit and/or vegetable salads and eat the salads daily. If you develop symptoms of heart rhythm disturbances, such as skipped beats, slow heart rate, rapid heart rate or chest pains, see your doctor immediately.

Selenium

As important as potassium is for saving lives from sudden death, so is selenium indispensable for preventing deaths of a different kind: those due to chronic degenerative diseases. Selenium is one of Nature's most important cancer-blocking agents. Studies have shown that cancer is far less prevalent in regions with high water and soil content of selenium than in regions where selenium is not found. In addition, cancer patients have lower blood and tissue levels of selenium than healthy individuals.

Selenium offers significant protection against heart disease as well. Recent studies document that individuals with low tissue levels of selenium are at a higher risk for heart attacks than those whose selenium levels are normal.

The protective effects of selenium are due largely to its potent antioxidant function. Antioxidants prevent the tissue damage which occurs as a result of oxidation. Thus, selenium helps stall the aging process and prevents the onset of diseases of civilization such as arthritis, diabetes, multiple sclerosis, lupus, heart disease, and cancer. In fact, researchers have discovered that selenium not only blocks the oxidative processes that lead to these diseases but also may reverse the damage after it occurs.

Selenium offers protection against heavy metal toxicity. It helps the body eliminate heavy metals by increasing the rate of their excretion in the urine and feces. Selenium is a particularly effective antidote for chronic mercury intoxication.

Selenium is a powerful immune enhancing agent. The ability of white blood cells to destroy invaders is greatly accelerated when it is supplemented in the diet. In addition, the production of the human body's crucial anti-allergy and anti-microbial proteins, the antibodies, is significantly enhanced as a result of selenium therapy.

This mineral's ability to strengthen immunity may be the explanation behind its anti-allergy action. Virtually all chronic allergy patients improve after increasing their dietary intake of selenium, regardless of the type of allergies from which they suffer.

Individuals who are chronically exposed to radiation require elevated dosages of supplemental selenium. Unfortunately, hundreds of thousands of Americans are being exposed to chronic radioactivity. A listing of such individuals includes x-ray technicians, nuclear power plant employees, uranium miners, nuclear waste disposal workers, individuals undergoing routine x-rays, dentists and dental technicians, radiologists, surgeons, chiropractors and chiropractic technicians, interns and residents, radiological nurses, food irradiation plant workers, clock and watch laborers who work with radium, podiatrists, video game enthusiasts, and computer operators.   Additionally, individuals living within a thirty mile radius of a nuclear plant are subjected to excessive radiation exposure.[10]

The selenium content of food depends entirely upon soil levels. Thus, it is difficult to produce a comprehensive listing of selenium-rich foods. However, the finest sources are fresh meats, vegetables, nuts, seeds, and mushrooms.   For instance, the selenium content of beef raised in South Dakota, a region rich in selenium, may be several times greater than beef raised in Indiana, a region where the soil is devoid of selenium.

It is truly the dilemma of modern man that food is only as healthy and nutrient-rich as the soil upon which it is grown. As little as two hundred years ago virtually all of the soil in the world could have been regarded as virgin.   However, commercial farming, with its emphasis on synthetic agri-chemicals, has devastated the health of the soil wherever it is practiced.   Thus, while certain vegetables, such as garlic, radishes, and turnips, are traditionally regarded as rich sources of selenium, this would hold true only if the vegetables were grown in selenium-rich soil. Furthermore, even if the soil is rich in selenium, commercial fertilizers and chemical treatments may prevent the absorption of selenium into plants.

Nearly one third of the states have selenium-deficient soil. Many of these states have such a high cancer incidence that they are known collectively as the *cancer belt*. This region includes primarily the states surrounding the Great Lakes: Wisconsin, Illinois, Indiana, Ohio, Michigan, and Western New York. Also included in the cancer belt are the

---

10. The heightened risk for cancer in those exposed to radiation from nuclear power plants is no longer an uncertainty. For instance, a recent study published in England documented a tenfold increase in leukemia in children fathered by nuclear power plant employees.

Canadian provinces of Manitoba, Ontario, and Quebec; the latter two border the northern edges of the Great Lakes. Additionally, numerous coastal states, such as Washington, Oregon, Maine, Massachusetts, Connecticut, Rhode Island, Vermont, New Jersey, the Carolinas, West Virginia, and Florida, have selenium-deficient soil. Individuals living in these regions should routinely supplement their diets with an organically bound form of selenium (e.g. selenium-kelp, seleno-methionine, or selenium-yeast).

Which of these apply to you?

1. tendency to be allergic to foods, drugs, or chemicals
2. premature aging
3. loss of skin elasticity (excessive wrinkling)
4. raised brownish lesions on the face, back, abdomen, or legs
5. infertility or low sperm count
6. increased susceptibility to yeast/fungal infections
7. acne
8. increased susceptibility to colds, flu, or other infections
9. hair loss
10. prostate problems
11. delayed wound healing
12. dermatitis and/or eczema
13. chronic urinary tract infections
14. Do you consume alcoholic beverages on a daily basis?
15. Do you live in a large city affected by heavy smog?
16. Are you developing an increasing number of moles and/or liver spots?
17. Do you suffer from cataracts and/or macular degeneration?
18. Do you have a history of asthma, hives, throat swelling, or other severe allergic reactions?

19. Do you have a history of coronary artery disease, cardiomyopathy (i.e. heart muscle degeneration), atherosclerosis, and/or high blood pressure?
20. Do you have arthritis affecting several joints?
21. Do you suffer from inhalant allergies such as hay fever, fume intolerance, and mold sensitivity?
22. Do you have silver fillings in your teeth?
23. Do you have a history of internal and/or external cancer?
24. Do you have chronic fungal infections?
25. Do you have hepatitis?
26. Do you suffer from insulin-dependent diabetes?
27. Do you live in one of the low-selenium states located in the cancer belt?
28. Are you exposed to heavy concentrations of toxic chemicals or heavy metals (mercury, silver, lead, etc.)?
29. Do you have pancreatitis?

Your Score ____

1 to 6 points *Mild selenium deficiency:* Selenium deficiency, even in a mild state, cannot be taken lightly. One reason is that selenium protects the human body from toxic chemical exposure, heavy metal overload, radiation, and excessive sunlight. However, equally important is the fact that even a modest decline in selenium levels results in a corresponding decline in immune function.

Organically bound selenium is the ideal supplemental source. In fact, it is the only type which can be consumed in the doses suggested herein. Avoid sodium selenite; it is toxic even in relatively small dosages. On a daily basis take 200 mcg of organically bound selenium. Vitamin E potentiates the action of selenium. Therefore, also take 400 I.U. of natural source vitamin E. Increase consumption of selenium-rich foods, particularly radishes, turnips, carrots, raw nuts, and seeds.

7 to 14 points *Moderate selenium deficiency:* Follow the previously mentioned advice and increase the dosage of selenium to 400 mcg daily. Reduce this dosage to 300 mcg daily after one month. In addition, increase your intake of vitamin E to a minimum of 1200 I.U. daily, as the extra vitamin E will help conserve selenium, preventing its destruction by noxious agents.

15 and above *Severe selenium deficiency:* Warning—prolonged selenium deficit increases the risks for a variety of serious diseases, particularly cancer, heart disease, and arthritis. Immune impairment and allergic diseases are also associated with selenium deficiency. Take 500 mcg of organically bound selenium each day. Curtail the consumption of alcoholic beverages and eliminate refined sugar, flour, and rice from the diet. Increase the intake of raw vegetables, nuts, seeds, and whole grains, particularly brown rice. Take 1600 I.U. of vitamin E and 3,000 mg of vitamin C daily. After one month reduce the dosage of selenium to 400 mcg per day. After 90 days take a maintenance level of 200 mcg daily. Do not take megadoses of inorganic selenium, since it may cause toxicity.

Silicon

More abundant in the body than iron or calcium, silicon has recently been decreed essential to human nutrition. It is essential for the development of all connective tissues, including the tendons, ligaments, arterial walls, skin, and bones. Furthermore, it assists in maintaining bone hardness as well as flexibility. In fact, joint damage, degeneration, and/or deformity are primary symptoms of silicon deficiency.

Silicon is the most abundant mineral found in the earth's crust. However, despite its abundance in soil and water, silicon deficiency is common in America. That is because this mineral is found in large quantities only in pure unprocessed foods and fresh unpolluted water. How many Americans have a diet rich in these?

Perhaps the most celebrated role of silicon in human nutrition relates to its importance in the maintenance of healthy connective tissues: skin, hair, nails, joints, and bones. This is one reason there is a surging interest within the cosmetic industry for lotions, creams, and shampoos containing silicon (in the form of silica) as a primary active ingredient. Top dietary sources of silicon include well water, bottled mineral water, garden-fresh vegetables, fresh milk products, fresh whole grains, organic liver, and fresh lean meats. Additionally, wild game and wild herbs are exceptionally rich in silicon.

Which of these apply to you?

1. brittle hair, split ends and/or nails
2. hair loss
3. thin hair
4. impaired wound healing
5. varicose veins
6. high blood pressure
7. dry flaky skin
8. brittle bones and/or osteoporosis
9. dermatitis, psoriasis, and/or eczema
10. skin which breaks open easily
11. chronic lower back pain
12. weak joints and/or ligaments
13. rapidly aging skin
14. loss of skin elasticity
15. joint swelling and/or deformity
16. poor circulation
17. eczema
18. Do you drink softened water on a regular basis?

19. Do you consume refined sugar on a daily basis?
20. Do you have a history of heart or circulatory disease?
21. Do you drink reverse osmosis or distilled water on a regular basis?
22. Do you have a history of a collagen disease such as scleroderma, rheumatoid arthritis, fibromyositis, or lupus?
23. Are you a diabetic?
24. Do you have chronic lung infections?
25. Do you suffer from premature graying of the hair?
26. Do you have osteoporosis (thinning of the bones)?

Your Score _____

1 to 6 points *Mild silicon deficiency:* Take 1,000 mg of organic silica daily. Avoid refined sugars. Drink mineral, tap (purified), or well water; distilled, softened, and reverse osmosis water are devoid of silicon.

7 to 14 points *Moderate silicon deficiency:* Take 2,000 mg of organic silica daily. Avoid distilled, reverse osmosis, or softened water and drink mineral water instead. Curtail the consumption of refined sugar and flour; increase the consumption of raw and/or unprocessed foods.

15 and above *Severe silicon deficiency:* A systemic deficiency of silicon increases the risks for heart disease, arthritis, osteoporosis, balding, eczema, psoriasis, and cancer. Take 3,000 mg of organic silica daily and follow the recommendations suggested for mild-moderate deficiencies. Curtail the consumption of refined sugars, alcoholic beverages, white flour, and other processed foods. Eat wild game as often as possible and consume several helpings each day of raw vegetables, nuts, and/or seeds.

Sodium

Much has been written in nutritional/medical circles about sodium, but it has largely been negative. This is unfortunate, since sodium is essential to human existence. Though it may be a surprise to many people, sodium is a necessary nutrient for the preservation of optimal health. Historians note that many centuries ago salt was so valuable that men traded it for its weight in gold. In contrast, the medical profession teaches that salt is dangerous and that the public should avoid it at all costs. While it is true that certain individuals are salt-sensitive and must curb their intake, the majority of Americans would suffer no ill effects by keeping salt in their diets.

The frequent prescription of the low sodium diet may, in fact, be dangerous. Sodium deficiency is surprisingly common in Americans. In certain individuals sodium deficiency becomes so extreme that blood levels dip below the normal range. This is a consequence of a condition known as the *Sodium Wasting Syndrome*. I discovered this syndrome in 1987 in Arlington Heights, Illinois, while treating patients in my clinic. Individuals with this condition lose sodium into the urine in large amounts and, despite an excess of sodium in the diet, ultimately become sodium deficient. They literally lose sodium as fast as they consume it. Such individuals are particularly vulnerable to the development of the deficiency when placed on sodium restricted diets. They may become so grossly deficient in this mineral that they develop a variety of symptoms seemingly so vague that doctors usually brush them off as "stress-induced" or "psychological." Yet, these patients are ill as a result of a lack of sodium, since this mineral is essential for maintaining such critical functions as the blood electrolyte balance, cardiac tone and pumping power, nerve firing, and digestive juice synthesis.

Sodium wasting is a significant health malady. This mineral exerts several critical functions within human tissues, and low blood levels of sodium must not be regarded lightly.

For instance, when sodium is wasted, there is also a decrease in tissue fluid. The latter phenomenon is known as volume depletion and is defined as a massive loss of fluid and electrolytes from the blood and cells. In other words, sodium is an anti-dehydrating agent.

Volume depletion is largely what happens in heat exhaustion and heat stroke. In this potentially fatal circumstance the loss of water as well as electrolytes, such as sodium bicarbonate, magnesium, and potassium, occurs. Ideally, treatment should include water and electrolyte replacement. In fact, drinking an excess of mineral-free water may precipitate heat exhaustion by a "washing out" effect, leading to a reduction in serum electrolyte levels. Thus, in the case of the sodium waster, dietary salt is necessary to help maintain fluid balance and prevent excessive loss of water from the tissues.

Low levels of sodium can be confirmed by blood testing. Indeed, it may be necessary to prescribe sodium as a therapeutic agent when blood levels are persistently low. I have frequently recommended that patients who suffer from the Sodium Wasting Syndrome use a heavy hand with the salt shaker (a good sea salt) and certainly should salt their food to taste without concern.

The majority of individuals with the Sodium Wasting Syndrome have developed it as a consequence of suffering from a chronic debilitating condition known as *adrenal insufficiency*. The adrenal glands produce the human body's sodium preserver, a hormone called *aldosterone*. This hormone "instructs" the kidneys to retain sodium by keeping it in the bloodstream and preventing it from being dumped into the urine. Without adequate amounts of aldosterone, millions of molecules of sodium are spilled into the urine every minute. Thus, salt must be continually replenished via the diet, although an additional approach would be to take aldosterone, a prescription drug.

However, the key to normalizing the sodium level is enhancing adrenal function through improved diet and nutritional supplementation. With improved adrenal function, sodium wasting is reduced or may be halted entirely.

Sea salt is preferable over table salt for several reasons. Table salt contains additives, including sugar (as dextrose) and aluminum. The aluminum prevents caking, and the sugar is probably added to make the taste of salt more appealing. In addition to being additive-free, sea salt contains a plethora of minerals besides sodium. Both sea salt and iodized table salt are rich sources of iodine. A very real concern is that sea salt may contain residues of toxic chemicals. To minimize this, purchase sea salt which is collected from regions other than the coastal United States. One of the best sources of sea salt is *Celtic Salt* from France. It is the least processed of all sea salts and retains an exceptionally high and diversified mineral content. Another option is land-derived salts. One of the finest is *Real Salt*, a pollutant-free salt extracted from an ancient seabed in Utah. Either of these quality salts may be ordered by calling 1-800-243-5242.

Which of these apply to you?

1. confusion and/or hallucinations
2. seizures
3. muscular weakness
4. lethargy and/or fatigue
5. lack of appetite
6. muscle cramps
7. headaches
8. excessive urination and/or urge to urinate from stress
9. cold weather causes urge to urinate
10. diarrhea
11. cold extremities
12. paranoia
13. psychotic behavior
14. low blood pressure
15. nausea and/or vomiting

16. dizziness
17. apathy
18. lack of thirst
19. Is your blood cholesterol level low?
20. Do you have a tendency to become dehydrated?
21. Do you adhere to a sodium-restricted diet?
22. Do you take diuretics on a daily or weekly basis?
23. Do you drink distilled and/or reverse osmosis water on a regular basis?
24. Do you crave salt or salty foods?
25. Have you been diagnosed with Addison's disease?
26. Do you exercise vigorously several times per week?
27. Are you unusually sensitive to heat, especially hot, humid weather, saunas, hot tubs, etc.?
28. Do you have difficulty digesting meat and other protein-rich foods?
29. Is your serum sodium low (below 139 mg/dl)?
30. Do you suffer from lack of concentration or memory loss?

Your Score ____

1 to 5 points *Mild sodium deficiency:* All that usually needs to be done at this stage is to increase the consumption of salt and salty foods.

6 to 11 points *Moderate sodium deficiency:* Individuals who score in this category and who adhere to a low sodium diet should begin adding sodium to their diets and use a heavy hand with the salt shaker. Take 1,000 to 2,000 mg of pantothenic acid daily, as this helps stimulate the synthesis of aldosterone, the adrenal hormone which helps conserve sodium. Be sure to eat salty snacks between meals and use salt in all cooking.

12 to 20 points *Severe sodium deficiency:* Fill 2 gelatin capsules with sea salt and take the salt capsules with every meal. Salt all foods to taste. Take 3,000 mg of pantothenic acid and 4,000 mg of vitamin C each day. In addition, be sure to consume plenty of foods rich in cholesterol; aldosterone is made from cholesterol. Take 3 capsules of Mexican yam extract three times daily.

21 and above *Extreme sodium deficiency:* Follow the previously mentioned recommendations for nutritional supplements. Fill 3 to 4 gelatin capsules with sea salt and liberally salt all foods. Eat salty snacks between meals such as salted roasted nuts, sunflower seeds, olives, and pickles. Be sure to eliminate all dietary sources of refined sugar, since sugar places stress upon the adrenal glands leading to a depletion of aldosterone stores. Take Mexican yam extract 4 capsules three times daily.

Note: The symptoms of sodium deficiency are vague. Therefore, it is possible to develop a number of these symptoms while having no gross deficiency of sodium. Certain individuals may be sensitive to sodium, particularly those suffering from hypertension, kidney disease, or fluid retention. Such individuals should not add large amounts of sodium to their diets. If you have a history of any of these diseases or if you are wary of consuming sodium, get a blood test called a SMAC, which includes a serum sodium level. If the level is normal or high-normal, use only moderate amounts of salt. If the level is below 140 (as milliliters per deciliter), sodium-wasting is likely. Levels below 138 confirm the diagnosis of the Sodium Wasting Syndrome. Sodium levels often improve or normalize as a result of nutritional therapy. Thus, the need for salt replacement may diminish. If your sodium level is low, have the level rechecked approximately 60 days after beginning this program. When the level normalizes, stop consuming supplemental salt; instead, use salt to taste.

Zinc

Zinc is one of the most heavily researched of all nutrients. It is perhaps most renowned for its role in immunity; even mild zinc deficiency leads to impairment of the immune response. For men zinc is known particularly as the anti-prostatitis nutrient.

Stress causes a rapid depletion of tissue zinc levels. Wounds and injuries fail to heal normally in the event of zinc deficiency. This is true of a wide range of injuries, including cuts, bruises, abrasions, bed sores, ulcers (internal and external), sprains, and fractures.

Surgical patients are vulnerable for developing zinc deficiency, and the post-surgical period is the worst time for this to occur. Such patients desperately need zinc for healing and for preventing post-surgical infections. A few surgeons have recognized this dilemma and are infusing zinc along with other critical nutrients by vein after surgery.

Not only do wounds heal slowly when zinc is deficient, but they are also highly likely to become infected. In zinc-deficient children minor cuts could result in pus-filled wounds or even sepsis (blood poisoning). Additionally, impetigo and various other staph infections, as well as acne, are correlated with poor zinc nutriture. Adults may suffer similar consequences. Individuals who repeatedly develop boils, infected cysts, fingernail bed infections (paronychia), and staph/strep infections are invariably zinc deficient. Further, individuals who suffer from repeated bouts of the flu, pneumonia, ear infections, tonsillitis, or sore throats, or who fail to recover rapidly after such infections, are in all likelihood severely deficient in zinc.

Molecularly, zinc is a rather large mineral. Less than 30% of the zinc ingested via food is absorbed into the blood. Absorption from zinc supplements may be as low as 5 to 10%.

The duodenum is the primary site of absorption. Absorption declines significantly in those suffering from digestive diseases, particularly those diseases affecting the upper portion of the small intestine. Thus, in individuals afflicted with duodenal ulcer, intestinal worms, giardia infection, grain allergies (gluten intolerance), and Crohn's disease, absorption is often minimal and extreme zinc deficiency usually occurs.

Certain drugs, notably alcohol, diuretics, cortisone, Tagamet, Zantac, and antacids, significantly impair zinc absorption. Ensminger states that alcohol may "precipitate a zinc deficiency by flushing...zinc out of the liver and into the urine."

Certain foods impair zinc absorption. Whole grains contain the zinc antagonist called phytic acid (pl. *phytates*). Beans and lentils contain certain fibrous compounds which destroy zinc. Because of the large concentration of phytates, plant protein, when ingested in large amounts, is one of the most common causes of zinc deficit. In particular, soy protein aggressively induces zinc deficiency. Soybeans are unusually rich in copper, which is a zinc antagonist. Thus, vegetarians who eat primarily soy as a protein source, frequently develop zinc deficiency.

Zinc is a crucial component of a wide range of human enzyme systems. Without zinc, the enzymes are rendered inoperable. Zinc-dependent enzymes control the following functions:

a) digestion of protein
b) fatty acid metabolism
c) sugar metabolism
d) bone deposition
e) skin cell formation synthesis
f) hair growth
g) sex hormone synthesis

h) insulin synthesis
i) thymic hormone synthesis

Zinc is rapidly destroyed when food is processed. Thus, only wholesome unprocessed food can be relied upon to provide adequate amounts of dietary zinc. As much as 80% of the zinc is lost when whole grains are refined. Similar losses result when fruits and vegetables are canned or frozen. However, organically grown produce and grains contain up to ten times the zinc as does commercially grown food. Top sources of zinc include crab, herring, liver, lobster, oysters, lamb, turkey, poppy seeds, caraway seeds, and whole grains.

Which of these apply to you?

1. lack of appetite or anorexia
2. lack of taste
3. white spots on the fingernails
4. reduced sperm count and/or infertility
5. lack of smell
6. chronic or recurrent ear infections
7. acne
8. slow growing hair and/or nails
9. increased susceptibility to colds, flu, or other infections
10. hair loss
11. prostate problems (prostatitis)
12. delayed wound healing
13. geographic tongue
14. growth impairment
15. light-colored pigment in the hair
16. dermatitis
17. blood sugar disturbances
18. dry and/or brittle hair
19. excessively dry or oily skin
20. sties on the eyelids
21. stretch marks

22. premature graying of the hair
23. irregular menstrual cycles (especially in teenagers)
24. impotence (lack of erection)
25. delayed sexual maturity
26. growing pains (or aching joints in teenagers)
27. sore or inflamed cracks in the skin at the fingertips
28. hangnails
29. chapped or split lips
30. recurrent vaginal yeast infections
31. delayed sexual maturation
32. growth impairment (stunted growth)
33. sensitivity of the eyes to light
34. enlarged facial pores
35. Do you consume refined sugars on a daily basis?
36. Do you consume alcoholic beverages on a daily or weekly basis?
37. Are you a diabetic?
38. Do you develop canker sores or other oral ulcerations?
39. Do you have a history of gout?
40. Do you consume large amounts of whole grains and/or grain brans on a daily basis?
41. Do you take diuretics on a daily or weekly basis?
42. Do you suffer from repeated bouts of chronic skin infections?
43. Do you suffer from recurrent urinary tract infections?
44. Does your skin sunburn easily or do you develop sun-induced rashes?
45. Do you have difficulty digesting meat or other protein-rich foods?
46. Do you have a history of detached retina or retinal bleeding?
47. Do you have macular degeneration?
48. Do you exercise vigorously on a daily basis?

49. Have you experienced prolonged periods of psychic stress?
50. Do you develop urinary tract infections frequently?
51. Do you suffer from duodenal ulcer, or have you had your duodenum removed?
52. Do you suffer from pancreatic disease?
53. Do you suffer from osteoporosis?
54. Do you have sclerosis and/or hepatitis?
55. Do you take cortisone on a daily or weekly basis?
56. Do you take birth control pills?
57. Do you take large amounts of supplemental calcium on a daily basis?

Your Score _____

1 to 7 points *Mild zinc deficiency:* Take a multiple vitamin-mineral tablet containing zinc and increase the consumption of zinc-rich foods.

8 to 16 points *Moderate zinc deficiency:* In addition to the multiple vitamin-mineral supplement take 30 mg of zinc daily. Consume zinc-rich foods on a daily basis. Avoid the brans of grains in order to reduce the consumption of phytates, which bind zinc and prevent its absorption. Curtail the consumption of all dietary sources of refined sugars and, if you drink alcohol regularly, quit.

17 to 29 points *Severe zinc deficiency:* Zinc deficiency greatly impairs immune response. Individuals suffering from this level of deficiency are vulnerable to the development of a variety of infections, particularly yeast infections, urinary tract infections, tuberculosis, influenza, and the common cold. Follow the previously mentioned measures and take 75 mg of zinc daily. After two months reduce this dosage to 50 mg daily. Alcohol, refined flour, and refined sugar should be

completely avoided. At this dosage be sure to take supplemental copper (4 mg per day).

30 and above *Extreme zinc deficiency:* Warning—zinc is essential to the synthesis of genetic material and is, therefore, required for cellular growth. Furthermore, protein synthesis throughout all tissues is dependent upon this mineral. Thus, at this level of deficiency cellular damage will occur. It is crucial to correct this zinc deficiency immediately. Moreover, further losses of zinc must be minimized. Avoid substances which deplete zinc, a category which includes alcohol, refined sugar, white flour, white rice, coffee, and certain drugs, notably diuretics and birth control pills. Increase the consumption of foods rich in zinc, being sure to include these foods in daily menus. However, avoid consuming excessive amounts of whole grains and grain fibers, such as wheat, corn, or oat bran, since they bind zinc and may induce a deficiency by preventing its absorption. In addition to dietary sources, take 75 to 100 mg of zinc daily. Because this is megadose therapy, be sure to take 2 mg of copper morning and night. The copper is needed because when zinc is taken in large doses, copper absorption is severely impaired. Thus, a secondary copper deficiency may result from prolonged megadose zinc therapy. Alcohol and medicinal diuretics are especially dangerous, since they aggressively flush zinc into the urine.[11]

---

11. To determine a zinc deficiency is quite easy. There is a nutritional zinc test called *Zinc Tally*. It is a liquid form of zinc, and, depending on the taste or lack of taste, this indicates the level of zinc sufficiency or deficiency. Zinc Tally may be found in many health food stores, or call Nutritional Supplement Service at (800) 243-5242.

Para Amino Benzoic Acid (PABA)

Para amino benzoic acid is actually a derivative of folic acid. However, as a separate substance it has important actions of its own. Research has found that PABA is exceptionally valuable for blocking the ill effects of sunlight on the skin. In fact, creams rich in PABA can be used to treat sunburn after it occurs, since PABA is a powerful antioxidant for stimulating tissue healing. It has also been discovered that PABA has an anti-graying action for the hair and not only prevents premature graying but may also actually restore hair to its original color. What's more, it plays an important role in the prevention of hair loss. Because of these functions, it may be regarded as the "healthy hair and skin" vitamin. PABA is found in the same food sources as folic acid.

Certain individuals may be allergic to PABA. This allergy often manifests as an intolerance to sunscreens containing PABA. If you are one of these PABA-sensitive individuals, internal consumption is contraindicated. In this instance the health benefits of PABA may be achieved through the use of folic acid, since this vitamin is closely related to PABA and possesses many of its functions.

Which of these apply to you?

1. premature graying of the hair
2. vitiligo (tiny white spots on the skin due to loss of pigment)
3. depression
4. chronic fatigue
5. chronic headaches
6. nervousness and/or irritability
7. skin rashes and/or dermatitis
8. hair loss
9. constipation

10. Do you take sulfa drugs for bacterial infections on a monthly, weekly, or daily basis?
11. Do you regularly take antibiotics (besides sulfa drugs)?
12. Do you sunburn easily?
13. Do you suffer from irritable bowel syndrome, ulcerative colitis, Crohn's disease, and/or celiac disease?
14. Have you had a portion of your intestines removed?
15. Do you have a history of autoimmune disease (thyroiditis, endometriosis, fibromyositis, polymyositis, diabetes, or lupus)?
16. Is your skin aging rapidly?
17. Do you suffer from an excessive amount of age or liver spots?
18. Are you constantly being exposed to radiation or x-rays?

Your Score _____

1 to 4 points *Mild PABA deficiency:* Take 200 mg of PABA daily and use sunscreens containing PABA.

5 to 10 points *Moderate PABA deficiency:* Be sure to use sunscreens containing PABA whenever you are exposed to the sun. Take 500 mg of PABA twice daily along with 2 mg of folic acid daily, since this helps conserve PABA.

11 and above *Severe PABA deficiency:* Take 1,000 mg of PABA twice daily. If you are suffering from vitiligo, severe graying of the hair and/or hair loss, increase the dosage to 3 grams (3000 mg) daily. If there is no response, try 5 grams of PABA and add 5 mg of folic acid. Use sunscreens containing PABA whenever you are exposed to the sun. Again, there is a word of caution. Individuals who react to PABA in sunscreens may also be sensitive to oral consumption: If you are reactive, quit all oral doses of PABA.

Amino Acids

Amino acids are a group of nutrients which are derived from proteins in our foods. They are a rather large group of compounds; over forty are known in Nature. This means that there is a greater number of amino acids than all the vitamins and minerals combined.

All proteins in the human body—enzymes, hair, skin, or the cells of the internal organs—consist of amino acids. They are truly the functional and structural building blocks of the human system. Thus, deficiencies of one or more amino acids could have a wide range of deleterious effects upon an individual's health status.

Many Americans, particularly children, teenagers, and the elderly, experience insufficient protein intake. This may lead to a condition known as *negative nitrogen balance*. Protein consists primarily of nitrogen, and, when the nitrogen level (in the form of amino acids) drops to a certain crucial point, negative nitrogen balance begins. This is manifested by a sort of cannibalistic state where the tissues utilize nitrogen from muscles and similar "non-essential" tissues in order to return the nitrogen balance to normal. Negative nitrogen balance may also be caused by the consumption of large quantities of refined sugar. The typical diet followed by teenagers, children, and many elderly individuals may contain as much as one-fourth to one-half cup of sugar per day. Think about it. A can of pop contains six to seven teaspoons of sugar; a few cookies, add another four or five teaspoons; a doughnut, add another seven teaspoons; a hamburger with special sauce, ketchup, and fries covered with ketchup, add three teaspoons (there is sugar in the bun, sauce, and ketchup); a chocolate malt, add 8 teaspoons. It doesn't take long to accumulate a quarter or even half cup.

The primary problem with excessive sugar intake is that high-quality protein-rich foods are being displaced by the sugary ones. However, there is an additional insidious factor:

sugar-induced protein damage. The refined sugar actually causes oxidative destruction of the amino acids within the body by a phenomenon known as *cross-linking*. Cross-linking is defined as a condition wherein cellular membranes become so damaged that they become hardened and stick together. Thus, the sugar is stiffening human tissues from the inside out and is greatly accelerating the aging process. It is wreaking havoc upon the cellular proteins and membranes, altering them from their flexible fluid-like state to a stiffened and, therefore, malfunctioning one. In essence, the cell membranes and proteins become functionally incompetent as a result of excessive sugar intake.

Sugar addicts frequently have high uric acid levels in their blood. Uric acid is a breakdown product of cellular nuclear material. What is the implication? Sugar is killing human cells.

Individuals who receive a significant percentage (25% or more) of their dietary calories from refined sugar are at the greatest risk for amino acid deficiency. Cooked sugar is worse, because the caramelization process increases the toxicity of the sugar. Additional high risk groups for protein deficiency are vegetarians and macrobiotic adherents. Their diets often omit the top sources of amino acids: meats, eggs, fish, and milk products.

The finest food source of amino acids is milk, which is a complete protein. Fresh milk, cottage cheese, and yogurt are the most readily available food sources for building a stable, healthy nitrogen balance. Unfortunately, tens of millions of Americans are allergic to cow's milk and/or products derived from it. However, goat's milk is an excellent alternative and is, in fact, more digestible than cow's milk. Yogurt is the most readily digested of all milk products, and the amino acids within it are efficiently absorbed into the bloodstream. Other excellent sources of protein/amino acids include brown rice, soybeans, alfalfa, spirulina, chlorella, and ground flax seed. Chlorella, spirulina, alfalfa, and ground flax seed are exceptionally valuable, since they are sources of raw (i.e. uncooked) amino acids. All of these products are available in quality health food stores.

Which of these apply to you?

1. mood swings
2. depression
3. anxiety and/or panic attacks
4. chronic fatigue
5. insomnia
6. weight loss
7. digestive disturbances
8. muscular weakness
9. chronic pain
10. impaired wound healing
11. heightened susceptibility to infection
12. diminished resistance to stress
13. nervousness and/or agitation
14. hair loss
15. slow growing hair and/or nails
16. brittle hair and/or nails
17. dry skin and/or hair
18. split ends
19. Do you drink one or more alcoholic beverages per day?
20. Were you a heavy drinker in the past?
21. Do you drink four or more cups of coffee per day?
22. Do you consume beverages or foods sweetened with NutraSweet on a daily basis?
23. Do you have a history of pancreatitis?
24. Do you have hypochlorhydria (low stomach acid)?
25. Have you had a portion of your stomach or intestines removed?
26. Do you have chronic anemia?
27. Do you have a history of panic disorder?
28. Do you fail to remember your dreams?

29. Do cuts or burns heal slowly?
30. Do you have reduced levels of protein in your blood (low BUN, albumin, globulin, creatinine, etc.)?

Your Score _____

1 to 6 points *Mild amino acid deficiency:* Take digestive enzymes (2 or 3 capsules with each meal) as an aid to protein digestion. Increase the intake of protein rich foods, especially highly digestible proteins such as chlorella, spirulina, bee pollen, eggs, raw nuts/seeds, and milk products.

7 to 12 points *Moderate amino acid deficiency:* Follow the previously mentioned advice plus take amino acids: 6 to 8 capsules of amino acid complex in the morning with a glass of juice (on an empty stomach). The sugar in the juice aids in amino acid absorption. An alternative would be to consume pre-digested protein supplements. Increase the dosage of digestive enzymes to 4 tablets/capsules with each meal. Eat fresh fish two or more times per week, since it is an excellent source of digestible protein.

13 to 19 points *Severe amino acid deficiency:* Follow the aforementioned advice. Additionally, take 50 mg each of B-6 and zinc, since protein digestion and synthesis cannot proceed without them. Take an additional 3 to 4 enzyme tablets one hour after meals. Try the Protein Shake recipe. Eat a couple of handfuls of raw nuts every day.

20 and above *Extreme amino acid deficiency:* Such an extreme in amino acid deficit requires aggressive correction. Increase the intake of protein-rich foods such as raw nuts/ seeds, bee pollen, ground flax seed, eggs, yogurt, and alfalfa meal. Take the following supplements:

- zinc - 30 mg twice daily
- B-6 - 50 mg twice daily
- digestive enzymes - 8 capsules twice daily (on an empty stomach with juice)
- bee pollen - one teaspoon with breakfast and an additional teaspoon with lunch
- chlorella - 15 (tiny) tablets with breakfast and an additional 15 with lunch

Bioflavonoids

Bioflavonoids are a unique class of natural chemicals found exclusively in fruits, vegetables, herbs, and other plants. Thousands of bioflavonoids exist in Nature, so many, in fact, that it is doubtful that researchers will ever be able to fully comprehend or quantify them. What's more, each plant has its own unique combination of bioflavonoids. For instance, alfalfa contains more than 40 different bioflavonoids, each of which possesses a separate chemical function.

Recently, bioflavonoids have been intensively studied because of their anti-inflammatory effects, since they possess powers similar to many drugs. One group of scientists found that bioflavonoids, when combined with enzymes and vitamin C, perform equally as well as a commonly prescribed anti-inflammatory drug in reducing swelling, pain, and inflammation. Relatively few bioflavonoids have been thoroughly studied, and even with this mere glimpse of knowledge researchers have become impressed at their potent therapeutic value in the treatment of disease. Familiar forms are rutin, hesperidin, catechin, and quercetin. Some examples of foods containing therapeutic bioflavonoids include:

Blueberries: contain bioflavonoids which prevent bruising, strengthen arteries, and enhance vision.

Cherries, strawberries, and grapes: contain a bioflavonoid (e.g. ellagic acid) which blocks the development of cancer and inactivates cancer-causing compounds.

Turmeric: contains bioflavonoids which reduce inflammation in the liver and aid in the treatment of liver diseases, including hepatitis and cirrhosis.

Ginger: contains bioflavonoids which block inflammation in the stomach, intestines, and liver as well as aid in the healing of damaged tissues within these organs.

Alfalfa: contains bioflavonoids which reduce inflammation in the lungs and joints, for instance, that which occurs in asthma, pneumonia, bronchitis, or arthritis.

Green cabbage: contains unique bioflavonoids which aid in the healing of internal ulcers, particularly stomach ulcers, and help prevent ulcer recurrence. Green cabbage juice is perhaps the most effective natural cure for internal ulcers. Other bioflavonoids in cabbage help block and/or reverse the toxic effects of nuclear radiation.

Citrus rind: contains bioflavonoids which reduce and/or eliminate inflammatory reactions in the joints. Citrus bioflavonoids also strengthen blood vessel walls and, thus, are effective in the treatment of nosebleeds, heavy periods, repeated abortions, bleeding gums, and easy bruising.

Bioflavonoids are found in all fruits, herbs, and vegetables. One method for determining the bioflavonoid content of a plant is the intensity of its color. Thus, red sweet peppers contain a greater number of bioflavonoids than green peppers, dark greens contain more than the light-colored iceberg lettuce, red onions contain a greater amount than yellow onions, dark bing cherries contain more than red cherries, etc. Additionally, fresh sun-ripened produce contains a richer bioflavonoid content than produce which is picked green and gas-ripened.

Recently, researchers discovered one of the most potent bioflavonoids ever. It is extracted from the Maritime pine tree in France. Pycnogenol, as it is called, is a highly effective antioxidant. Its antioxidant properties are significantly more potent than either vitamin C or vitamin E. It is beneficial in the treatment of a variety of conditions, including spider veins, liver spots, cholesterol deposits, back pain, arthritis, asthma, prostate problems, eczema, fibromyalgia, and inflammation. Excellent food sources of bioflavonoids include alfalfa, turmeric, red peppers (sweet and hot), bing cherries, red cabbage, tangerines, oranges, grapefruit, lemons, limes, alfalfa, strawberries, raisins, and black currants.

Which of these apply to you?

1. easy bruising
2. bleeding gums
3. nosebleeds
4. inflammation and/or swelling of the joints
5. swollen extremities
6. varicose and/or spider veins
7. heavy menstrual bleeding
8. retinal hemorrhages
9. repeated miscarriages
10. tendency to form blood clots
11. blood in the urine
12. hemorrhoids
13. glaucoma
14. fragile blood vessels (blood vessels which burst easily)
15. arthritis
16. fever blisters
17. petechiae (tiny red blood spots on the skin)

18. failing vision
19. blood in the stool
20. Do you have a history of coronary artery disease or hardening of the arteries?
21. Have you had blood clots in the veins?
22. Have you had numerous miscarriages?
23. Have you suffered a stroke, or do you have a significant family history of stroke?
24. Do you have a history of stomach and/or duodenal ulcers?
25. Do you have a significant family history of stroke and/or have you experienced a stroke?
26. Do you avoid consuming fresh fruits and/or vegetables?
27. Do you consume aspirin, Motrin, or other anti-inflammatory drugs on a daily or weekly basis?
28. Do you suffer from failing vision?
29. Do you suffer from shingles or genital herpes outbreaks?

Your Score _____

1 to 5 points *Mild bioflavonoid deficiency:* Take 1,000 mg of citrus bioflavonoids daily. In addition, consume foods and spices rich in bioflavonoids.

6 to 13 points *Moderate bioflavonoid deficiency:* Take 1,500 to 2,000 mg of citrus bioflavonoids daily. Take also 30 mg of pycnogenol twice daily. On a regular basis eat large helpings of fruits and vegetables rich in bioflavonoids.

14 and above *Severe bioflavonoid deficiency:* A systemic deficiency of bioflavonoids increases the risks for bleeding disorders such as nosebleeds, easy bruising, bleeding ulcers, and petechiae (ruptured capillaries). Take 3,000 mg of citrus bioflavonoids daily. Take 60 mg of pycnogenol twice daily. In addition, take 3 to 5 capsules of bee propolis each day, the richest known source of bioflavonoids. Also take vitamin C;

it works synergistically with the bioflavonoids to strengthen blood vessels and reduce inflammation (3,000 mg daily). Vitamin E helps obviate bleeding tendencies by normalizing blood clotting (take 1200 I.U. daily).

Enzymes (digestive)

Enzymes are complex protein molecules. They function to speed the various chemical reactions occurring within the human body. Incredibly, billions of enzyme molecules are synthesized every day by our bodies, primarily in the liver, pancreas, and small intestine.

Enzyme deficiency is extremely common in the United States as well as in other Western countries. In this syndrome the pancreas, the gland responsible for the synthesis of digestive enzymes, fails to produce the appropriate amount of enzymes for food to be digested optimally. This is largely a result of enzyme burnout from the prolonged consumption of processed and chemically contaminated foods.

The pancreas synthesizes the vast majority of the enzymes. Unfortunately, pancreatic enzyme depletion is common in Americans and is largely the result of poor diet. Nearly 80% of the calories consumed by Americans today come from processed foods. Furthermore, there are well over 6,000 synthetic chemicals which are "legally" added to food. This does not include pesticide and herbicide residues; the majority of commercial food contains detectable levels of them. It is no wonder that pancreatic disease is common in America today. The pancreas is a delicate organ and is readily damaged by toxic insults. However, it may take a number of years before it finally collapses as a result of chemical toxicity, sugar overload, alcoholism, and/or nutritional deficiency.

A number of substances commonly found in the American diet induce pancreatic damage. These substances

162

include coffee, alcohol, tobacco smoke, artificial sweeteners, food preservatives, food dyes, drugs, sulfites, MSG, pesticides, herbicides, and refined sugar. The latter is the most ubiquitous anti-pancreatic agent. A high-sugar diet causes a significant reduction in pancreatic enzyme output. The long-term ill effects on the pancreas are well known: hypoglycemia and, ultimately, diabetes—perhaps even cancer.

Diabetes afflicts millions of Americans, and hundreds of thousands of children and adolescents are included in its victims. Ironically, diabetes is entirely preventable by curtailing the intake of refined sugar early in life.

Sugar is only one of many culprits. Artificial sweeteners may in some respects exhibit an even greater degree of toxicity to the pancreas than refined natural sugars. Studies document that NutraSweet essentially stops the pancreas from producing enzymes. After only a few doses, the equivalent of that found in a half dozen cans of pop, enzyme production comes to a screeching halt.

A deficiency in digestive enzymes can result in a number of symptoms, most of them related directly to digestion. However, digestive enzymes are involved in a variety of other functions, including protein synthesis, antimicrobial activity, and cellular cleanup, the latter being a sort of garbage collector/processor function.

Enzymes are found in all foods, but they are destroyed by heat. Thus, raw and lightly cooked foods are the only significant dietary sources.

Which of these apply to you:

1. excessive gas
2. fullness and/or bloating after meals
3. poorly formed stools
4. constipation
5. greasy, pale, or gray stools that float

6. chronic heartburn
7. undigested food particles in stool
8. chronic diarrhea
9. colitis and/or irritable bowel syndrome
10. eczema and/or psoriasis
11. hives and/or other severe allergic reactions
12. lack of appetite
13. white spots on the fingernails
14. ridges on the fingernails
15. slow growing nails and/or hair
16. hair loss
17. stomach or bowel pain after eating
18. fatigue and/or somnolence after eating
19. rectal burning
20. Do you have a significant family history of diabetes, or do you suffer from diabetes?
21. Do you have hypochlorhydria (low stomach acid)?
22. Do you have a history of pancreatitis?
23. Do you consume on a daily basis one or more servings of foods/beverages containing artificial sweeteners?
24. Do you have a history of stomach or intestinal cancer?
25. Do you smoke and/or use chewing tobacco?
26. Is your diet high in refined sugar?
27. Do you consume alcoholic beverages on a daily basis?
28. Do you eat processed foods or fast foods on a daily basis?
29. Do you eat mostly cooked foods?
30. Do you avoid eating raw fruit and vegetables?
31. Are you a ravenous eater, or do you eat excessively fast?
31. Do you drink five or more cups of coffee per day?
32. Do you have mucous in your stool?

Your Score _____

1 to 7 points   *Mild enzyme deficiency:* Increase the consumption of enzyme-rich raw fruits and vegetables. Take 3 capsules of papaya enzymes with all meals, particularly

high protein meals. Try also a digestive enzyme supplement such as Formula #416 (see Appendix C) with all meals, especially those consisting of cooked foods. Reduce your consumption of sugar, white flour, and/or alcohol.

8 to 17 points *Moderate enzyme deficiency:* In addition to eating raw foods take digestive enzymes, zinc, and vitamin B-6. Both zinc and B-6 stimulate enzyme synthesis in the pancreas. Take 3 to 4 capsules of digestive enzymes with every meal along with an additional 2 to 3 capsules one hour after meals. Curtail the consumption of NutraSweet and saccharin. Strictly avoid refined sugar as well as alcohol.

18 and above *Severe enzyme deficiency:* At this level of deficiency protein digestion and absorption is severely impaired. Aggressive treatment with digestive aids is indicated. In addition to the previous dietary recommendations follow this enzyme treatment regimen:

- With meals: 4 to 6 capsules of papaya enzymes and 4 capsules non-porcine pancreatin
- One hour after meals: 3 capsules of papaya enzymes and 3 capsules of non-porcine pancreatin
- Two hours after meals: 2 capsules of papaya enzymes and 2 capsules of non-porcine pancreatin

Coenzyme Q-10 (Co-Q-10)

Coenzyme Q-10 is one of the most unique of all nutrients. Technically, it fails to meet the criteria of a vitamin, yet, it is essential to life. When tissue levels of co-Q-10 fall to certain levels (25% of normal), death results. Co-Q-10 is produced in the body, but dietary intake represents a significant source. It is found widespread in foods, for which reason it was originally named "ubiquinone" (from the term *ubiquitous*).

One of coenzyme Q-10's main functions is the production of intracellular energy. In the case of humans the primary fuel produced on a cellular level is *ATP*, or *adenosine triphosphate*. This energy source is the basis of life, since all cellular reactions require and consume it. Thus, due to its role in energy production, coenzyme Q-10 is of crucial importance for organs with rapid metabolic rates such as the heart, thyroid gland, adrenal glands, kidneys, and lungs.

Coenzyme Q-10's role in cardiac function has received the greatest attention among researchers. In fact, it was originally extracted from heart tissue (bovine hearts), the richest known source of this nutrient. During the 1950s and 1960s researchers discovered that animals which developed co-Q-10 deficiency died of heart failure. The hearts would enlarge in size, and the pumping power decreased dramatically. When the diets were supplemented with co-Q-10, the cardiac size and function returned to normal. The next step was to test the effectiveness of co-Q-10 on humans suffering from a similar condition: congestive heart failure. The scientists discovered that co-Q-10 worked equally well for humans with heart disease and completely reversed the pathology in a number of instances. Further research documented a powerful role in the treatment of hypertension, heart rhythm disturbances, angina pectoris, and coronary heart disease. In all cases the diseased hearts of cardiac patients, particularly those with congestive heart failure, showed a measurable decline in co-Q-10 levels from the norm. Co-Q-10 is also of exceptional value in the treatment of cardiomyopathy, a condition which leads to degeneration of the heart muscle.

A number of other organs/tissues become diseased when co-Q-10 levels decline. They include the majority of internal organs, for instance the brain, liver, lungs, and kidneys, as well as visible organs such as the skin and gums. The gums are one of the most metabolically active tissues in the body and, thus, their need for co-Q-10 is exceptionally high. When co-Q-10 levels fall below a critical point, the gums degenerate. This is manifested by a lack of growth, recession, and an inability to adhere to the teeth. This recession causes the gums to become vulnerable to infection (pyorrhea).

Coenzyme Q-10 is similar chemically to vitamin E. The consequence of this similarity is perhaps best illustrated by the fact that many of the symptoms of vitamin E deficiency can be corrected by taking co-Q-10. Furthermore, vitamin E enhances the function of coenzyme Q-10. Thus, the two should always be taken in unison.

Coenzyme Q-10 is found in such a wide variety of foods that it is feasible to list only its richest sources: animal hearts and kidneys. Currently, virtually all coenzyme Q-10 available on the market is produced via microbial synthesis. This means that co-Q-10 supplements are natural extracts rather than being artificially produced in a laboratory from petrochemicals.

Which of these apply to you?

1. muscular weakness
2. heart rhythm disturbances
3. delayed wound healing
4. enlarged heart
5. morbid obesity
6. chronic unrelenting fatigue
7. bleeding gums and/or pyorrhea
8. receding gums
9. high blood pressure
10. chronic kidney disease
11. increased susceptibility to infections
12. chronic gum infections (pyorrhea)
13. foul breath
14. muscular atrophy
15. accelerated aging of the skin
16. Do you avoid eating fatty fish?

17. Do you have a difficult time initiating weight loss even while dieting?
18. Do you have an aversion/intolerance to exercise, or do you feel ill after exercising?
19. Do you have an immune deficiency disorder?
20. Do you have a history of angina pectoris and/or coronary artery disease?
21. Do you have a history of congestive heart failure?
22. Do you have asthma?
23. Do you avoid eating red meats and poultry?
24. Do you have chronic lung infection?
25. Do you smoke one-half pack or more of cigarettes daily?
26. Do you have shortness of breath after exertion?
27. Do you experience severe muscle pain, particularly after exercising?

Your Score _____

1 to 4 points *Mild coenzyme Q-10 deficiency*: Take 50 to 75 mg of co-Q-10 daily along with 400 I.U. of vitamin E. Avoid processed foods.

5 to 12 points *Moderate coenzyme Q-10 deficiency:* As tissue levels of coenzyme Q-10 begin to decline, the human body becomes vulnerable to the onset of rapid aging and degenerative disease. Protect yourself from rapid aging by consuming coenzyme Q-10 preventively. Take a minimum of 150 mg daily along with 800 I.U. of vitamin E. Reduce alcohol consumption and avoid refined vegetable oils.

13 and above *Severe coenzyme Q-10 deficiency*: Warning— severe coenzyme Q-10 deficiency may result in potentially life-threatening diseases such as congestive heart failure, asthma, emphysema, morbid obesity, and coronary artery disease. Take 200 mg of co-Q-10 daily. If you score greater than 18, take 300 mg daily. Eat beef or lamb hearts from

organically raised animals cooked lightly (medium or medium rare) three to five times weekly. Avoid all dietary sources of refined sugar as well as refined and/or hydrogenated oils. The refined oils oxidize or "use up" the co-enzyme Q-10 found in the body. Be sure to take 1200 I.U. of vitamin E daily. Additionally, if you have symptoms of congestive heart failure, asthma, or coronary artery disease, seek medical care immediately.

Essential Fatty Acids

Fat is a subject of much research and discussion in the field of nutrition. Mostly, the term conjures up negative thoughts in our minds. "Stay away from fats if you wish to avoid the major killers and remain healthy," we are told. While this may be true of certain fats, avoiding the essential fatty acids could prove dangerous. This is because these fats cannot be produced in the body and are required for the maintenance of the basic processes of existence. Without them, a variety of illnesses develop. The essential fatty acids are required for the synthesis of the cells of every organ in the body. In addition, hormone, protein, prostaglandin, and neurotransmitter synthesis are also dependent upon essential fatty acids. A list of the ailments which have been associated with essential fatty acid deficiency includes:

- eczema, dermatitis, and psoriasis
- lupus
- seborrheic dermatitis
- hair loss
- heart disease and hardening of the arteries
- diabetes
- arthritis
- senility
- Crohn's disease and irritable bowel syndrome
- acne
- asthma and emphysema
- Sjogren's syndrome

- cancer
- alcoholism
- Infertility
- adrenal insufficiency

A little-known fact is that the brain, when the weight of water is removed, consists primarily of fat. It possesses a dramatic need for essential fatty acids in order to function normally. What's more, whenever tissues within the brain, spinal cord, or the peripheral nerves are damaged, the need of the nervous system for essential fatty acids multiplies exponentially. In fact, the need is so great that the body will, figuratively speaking, "steal" fatty acids from other tissues in order to maintain the nervous system's requirements.

The saying that a person's brain is "shriveled up" may be literally true in the case of certain degenerative diseases of the brain, *many of which are caused by a prolonged deficiency of essential fatty acids*. The fatty acids are involved in moisture retention within the brain cells, and, in the event of deficiency a measurable reduction in the weight of the brain occurs. Naturally occurring fats which are required for nervous system function include linoleic acid, linolenic acid, lecithin, EPA/DHA (abbreviations for fish oils), and cholesterol. Mental symptoms which may arise in the event of severe essential fatty acid deficiency include:

- attention deficit
- violent behavior
- mania
- memory loss
- autism and/or retardation
- anxiety/depression
- headaches
- seizures

Essential fatty acids occur in tiny amounts in a variety of foods. The richest sources are nuts, seeds, and certain grains, notably fresh whole wheat, barley, oats, corn, and rice. Soybeans are also an excellent source. However, the top food source is flax seed, which contains a high percentage of lino*lenic* acid. This latter oil is difficult to procure in the American diet, which contains an excess of lino*leic* acid.

170

Other excellent sources of essential fatty acids include the oils extracted from the seeds of the primrose, hemp, caraway, black currant, and borage plants.

Food oils, such as those found in supermarkets, are traditionally regarded as top dietary sources of essential fatty acids. However, this is true only of those oils processed by cold-pressing methods. Commercial oils contain such a large number of contaminants and are so heavily processed that they can no longer be regarded as optimal sources.

Which of these apply to you?

1. dry, flaky skin
2. dryness or cracks behind the ears
3. brittle hair and/or fingernails
4. acne
5. enlarged facial pores
6. growth impairment
7. dry or oily hair
8. eczema/psoriasis/dermatitis
9. chronic diarrhea
10. alopecia (patchy hair loss)
11. nosebleeds
12. bleeding gums
13. easy bruising
14. dry patches of scaly skin on the face and/or nose
15. patches of hair which are unmanageable (stick up on end)
16. split ends
17. poor or delayed recovery from injuries
18. intolerance to or slow recovery from exercise
19. delayed wound healing
20. tingling in the arms and legs
21. lips which are constantly chapped
22. attention deficit disorder (poor attention span)
23. asthma
24. loss of appetite

25. gritty feeling in or dryness of the eyes
26. irritability and/or nervousness
27. PMS (especially painful menstrual cramps, bloating, and/or sore breasts)
28. sensation of dryness of the mouth and throat, especially when speaking
29. lack of tearing
30. obesity
31. unexplained weight loss
32. Do you take aspirin, Motrin, Indocin, Feldene, Naprosyn, or similar anti-inflammatory drugs on a daily or weekly basis?
33. Do you consume margarine on a daily or weekly basis?
34. Do you drink alcohol on a daily or weekly basis?
35. Do you consume refined sugars on a daily or weekly basis?
36. Do you have a history of repeated miscarriages?
37. Do you have Sjogren's syndrome and/or lupus?
38. Do you have emphysema and/or other chronic lung diseases?
39. Do you have Crohn's disease and/or irritable bowel?
40. Do you suffer from chronic joint pain (arthritis)?
41. Do you have a history of sluggish kidneys, chronic kidney disease, and/or bladder infections?
42. Do you have dementia, senility, Alzheimer's disease, and/or Parkinson's disease?
43. Do you have a history of ovarian cysts and/or fibrocystic breast disease?
44. Are you a diabetic?
45. Are you a tobacco smoker?
46. Do you have a history of prostate problems?
47. Do you take cortisone or prednisone on a daily or weekly basis?
48. Do you have a history of infertility or impotence?

172

49. Do you follow a very low fat diet?

50. Do you take cholesterol-lowering medicines?

Your Score ____

1 to 8 points *Mild essential fatty acid deficiency*: Take 2 to 4 capsules of primrose oil daily.   Use ground flax seed in recipes or as a topping on cereals, yogurt, or ice cream. Be sure to read all labels and avoid all foods containing hydrogenated and/or partially hydrogenated oils. These oils destroy the essential fatty acids.

9 to 18 points *Moderate essential fatty acid deficiency*: Take 8 capsules of primrose oil daily.   Add to this 3 heaping tablespoons of ground flax taken in juice, milk, or water. Do not consume commercial oils of any type. Take supplemental zinc, vitamin B-6, riboflavin, and magnesium on a daily basis.

19 to 27 points *Severe essential fatty acid deficiency*: The consumption of alcohol and other substances which destroy essential fatty acids must be curtailed immediately. Remove all refined sugars and oils from the diet. Consume only pure cold-pressed oils. Take 12 capsules of primrose oil daily in addition to 6 tablespoons of ground flax seed.

An additional source of essential fatty acids is hemp seed oil, which is made from the edible seed of the cannabis (marijuana) plant.   It is free of all hypnotic/intoxicating chemicals or effects.   This seed is consumed by various animals and birds and has been used since ancient times as a source of food. The oil contains an excellent distribution of critical essential fatty acids, including linoleic acid, linolenic acid, and gamma linolenic acid. Take 1 or 2 tablespoons daily.

Additionally, take vitamin B-6 (50 mg), zinc (50 mg), vitamin C (200 mg), vitamin E (800 I.U.), and magnesium (800 mg), since all of these are required for optimal utilization of essential fatty acids. Lipase, a fat-digesting enzyme, is also recommended for those who have poor fat assimilation.

28 and above   *Extreme essential fatty acid deficiency*: Prolonged deficiency of essential fatty acids is a serious concern, since the function of all organ systems is dependent upon them.   The earliest signs are manifested by skin disorders, as the skin is a barometer of essential fatty acid nutriture.   As the deficiency deepens, malfunction of the internal organs occurs, which may be represented by cellular degeneration, internal bleeding, and even cell death.

To correct this condition strictly avoid all dietary sources of refined, deep fried, and/or hydrogenated oils (see pages 184 to 192).   In addition, take 14 capsules of primrose oil, 6 capsules of lecithin, and 8 tablespoons of ground flax seed every day.   Supplement the diet with the nutrients necessary to stimulate fatty acid metabolism: B-6 (100 mg), vitamin C (3,000 mg), zinc (50 mg), magnesium (1,000 mg), vitamin E (1200 I.U.), and lipase (400 mg).

Individuals who score greater than 38 points should take 250 mg of B-6 and 75 mg of zinc daily.   At this zinc dosage be sure to take 4 mg of copper daily.   In addition, increase the dosage of primrose oil to twenty capsules daily.   These dosages may be reduced as soon as improvement is noted.

Lactobacillus Insufficiency Quiz

Lactobacillus cannot be classified as a nutrient. However, for the purposes of this discussion it may be regarded as an essential dietary/nutritional component, since, like nutrients, a deficiency of lactobacillus can develop, and it can be taken supplementally. The term lactobacillus defines a family of bacteria useful in the maintenance of optimal health and the prevention of disease. Several types of lactobacilli exist, including Lactobacillus acidophilus, Lactobacillus bifidus, Lactobacillus Caucasus, and Lactobacillus bulgaricus. These bacteria occur naturally in a variety of foods, although fermented milk products and sauerkraut are the richest sources.

Normally, these organisms are the predominant ones in the human intestine, existing in astronomically high numbers (several billion every few inches of bowel). However, in disease states and general ill health their numbers decline dramatically. The fact is millions of Americans suffer from lactobacillus deficiency. Why is the deficiency so common? Lactobacillus organisms are delicate creatures and are readily destroyed by noxious chemicals, particularly chlorine. Virtually everyone in the USA drinks chlorinated water. Chlorine is a potent oxidizing agent. In more familiar jargon it kills bacteria by "bleaching" them to death, leading to a gradual decline in bowel lactobacillus counts. Secondly, antibiotics wreak havoc upon lactobacillus organisms. A single course of antibiotics decimates bowel microbes, killing the intestinal flora by the billions. This leads to the overgrowth of certain organisms, such as Candida and others, which are resistant to antibiotics. The problem is that these organisms are pathogens, that is they are disease-causing. Antibiotics create this disastrous effect whether taken in drug form or consumed in food. Thus, eating antibiotic-laced meats, milk products, fish, and poultry leads to an insidious decline in the number of lactobacillus organisms within the body.

The lactobacillus count in the bowel/vagina is a predictor for an individual's vulnerability to certain diseases. This is because these bacteria, descriptively known as the friendly flora, inhibit the growth of disease-causing pathogens.

Diseases associated with a deficiency of lactobacillus include:

- psoriasis
- eczema
- lymphoma
- high cholesterol
- hepatitis
- chronic candidiasis
- irritable bowel syndrome
- diverticulitis
- seborrheic dermatitis
- acne
- heart disease
- ulcerative colitis
- stomach acid
- intestinal parasites
- lupus
- colon cancer

Lactobacillus organisms are found in small quantities within and/or on a variety of vegetables, grains, and fruits. However, they are found in large quantities only in fermented foods. Top food sources include yogurt, kefir, kefir cheese, quark, tempeh, and sauerkraut.

Which of these apply to you?

1. intestinal gas
2. bloating after meals
3. constipation
4. diarrhea
5. hard pebble-like stools
6. mucous in the stool
7. foul-smelling stools
8. hemorrhoids
9. easy bruising
10. recurrent nosebleeds
11. psoriasis and/or eczema
12. seborrhea of the scalp
13. indigestion and/or heartburn
14. Do you take antibiotics on a daily, weekly, or monthly basis?
15. Do you often eat commercial meat, poultry, and/or fish?

16. Do you rarely or never eat fermented milk products?
17. Were you, as a baby, bottle fed instead of breast fed?
18. Do you have a history of chronic candidiasis?
19. Are you unusually vulnerable to the development of intestinal flu and/or food poisoning?
20. Do you have ulcerative colitis, irritable bowel syndrome, or Crohn's disease?
21. Do you drink chlorinated water?
22. Do you have a history of diverticulitis or diverticulosis?

Your Score ____

1 to 4 points *Mild lactobacillus deficiency*: Increase the consumption of fermented milk products and yogurt. Eat at least one serving every day for one or two months. If you are allergic to milk products, take instead 2 capsules of Lactobacillus acidophilus and/or bifidus with every meal.

5 to 13 points *Moderate lactobacillus deficiency*: In addition to the yogurt take Lactobacillus acidophilus and/or bifidus supplements (1 or 2 capsules with meals). Curtail the consumption of commercially raised meats, opting instead for meats free of antibiotics and hormones. Avoid taking antibiotics, except for medical emergencies.

14 and above *Severe lactobacillus deficiency*: Consume large amounts of fermented milk products, for instance, three or four cups of yogurt daily. Take acidophilus and/or bifidus supplements, 3 capsules three times daily (with meals). Have your doctor take you off all antibiotics, topical and/or oral. Drink purified or mineral water instead of tap water or purchase a water treatment unit which removes chlorine.

The Water Deficiency (Dehydration) Quiz

Water is the basis of life. Up to 75% of the weight of the human body consists of water. It is the most crucial of all nutrients for survival. A human being can live for weeks without food but only for days without water.

Despite the fact that water is conveniently available in America, dehydration is just as common here as it is in many other regions of the world. This is largely because Americans often fail to make a conscious effort to consume water on a daily basis. There is another reason: essential fatty acid deficiency. The fatty acids act as a type of cellular glue, keeping cell membranes tightly fixed against each other. As such, essential fatty acids prevent excessive fluid losses, particularly from the skin. Individuals with severe essential fatty acid deficiency often become dehydrated, even if their fluid intake is normal.

There is yet another problem: water quality. Because of the concerns about water pollution and the toxicity of chlorine/fluoride, many individuals avoid drinking tap water, even though they might be thirsty. There is no easy solution for this dilemma. Keeping plenty of high quality bottled water near at hand is one method that would prevent dehydration. Tap water purifiers are yet another solution for making your water "consumable." Filtration drinking straws are another option. Some of these straws are capable of filtering up to 35 gallons of water and are ideal for use in traveling.

It is possible to consume too much water. In such an instance the body may be described as becoming "waterlogged." While relatively rare, the condition does arise occasionally in hospitalized patients receiving IV fluids. During my internship a surgical patient nearly died from water intoxication. She received an excess of IV fluids, which washed the electrolytes out of her body. The result was the patient developed seizures and slipped into a comatose state. She was subsequently "brought back to life" by infusing a concentrated salt solution.

Water poisoning also occurs in certain well-meaning fanatics. Such individuals often feel the need to "flush" poisons out of their bodies and may consume inordinate amounts of water—gallons—on a daily basis. Certain of these individuals consume purified water, such as distilled or reverse osmosis, which further depresses the electrolyte count.

Which of these apply to you?

1. chronic constipation
2. hemorrhoids
3. dry mouth and/or eyes
4. dry skin
5. dry nasal membranes
6. dry or chapped lips
7. urinate 3 times or less per day
8. leathery skin
9. tendency to get shocked by static electricity
10. varicose veins
11. Do you drink large amounts of coffee (more than 3 cups per day)?
12. Do you drink large amounts of beer (2 or more beers per day)?
13. Do you avoid drinking water, and/or do you consume less than 2 glasses of water per day?
14. Do you drink large amounts of tea (3 or more cups) on a daily basis?
15. Do you take diuretics on a daily or weekly basis?
16. Do you have dark colored and/or foul smelling urine?
17. Do you have recurrent urinary tract infections?
18. Do you have a history of kidney stones?

Your Score _____

1 to 4 points *Mild dehydration*: This condition is easily rectified; simply increase fluid consumption by drinking six to eight 8-ounce glasses of water per day. Avoid substances possessing diuretic actions such as tea, coffee, or water pills.

5 to 9 points *Moderate dehydration*: Increase fluid consumption by drinking six to eight 8-ounce glasses of water per day. Additionally, take essential fatty acids: 8 capsules of primrose oil or one tablespoon of cold-pressed flax seed or hemp seed oil each day. Avoid all diuretics.

10 and above *Severe dehydration*: Warning—prolonged dehydration may result in damage to the internal organs, particularly the kidneys. Drink at least eight large glasses of water per day and take essential fatty acids: 12 capsules of primrose oil or 2 tablespoons of flax oil or hemp oil daily. Curtail the consumption of coffee, tea, and alcohol. See your doctor if you are taking diuretics and request that he/she reduce the dosage or preferably eliminate the drug(s).

Section II

The Dietary Tests

Many people think they are eating right, but they are not. For instance, some people believe that by substituting margarine for butter they are eating right. Others believe that eating pasta on a regular basis is eating right. Still others think that they can eat junk food "once in a while," since they eat fruit, vegetables, and other wholesome foods on a regular basis. However, people with the latter attitude usually eat prodigious amounts of junk food. Vegetarians believe they are eating right. Yet, they are usually deficient in a number of nutrients as a result of their vegetarian diet. Macrobiotic adherents are also convinced they are eating right, often believing that their program is fit for all. Yet, all too often they suffer from a variety of nutritional deficiencies similar to those seen in vegetarians.

It is difficult to eat right in America. There is little good food in grocery stores. Organic produce is virtually impossible to find in most regions. Instead, the food that is available is full of chemicals and low in nutrients. As a result, the majority of Americans are eating all manner of junk and devitalized foods. Are pastries, TV dinners, potato chips, cookies, crackers, white bread, deep fried foods, preserved meats, canned vegetables, white rice, pasta, ice cream, pop, candy and similar nutritionally depleted foods still on your menu? None of these items can be defined as being wholesome fresh foods. Yet, these types of foods are the primary ones found in grocery stores as well as fast-food restaurants.

The preparation of the dietary tests required that I make several trips to the grocery store. I analyzed the ingredients of the various packaged foods, in other words, everything but fresh produce, milk products, and meats. These grocery store items were checked for their content of a variety of food components and additives. Remarkably, the majority of the food on supermarket shelves contained sugar. It is not the naturally occurring kind such as the sugar of an apple or the malt of a grain. Incredibly, of the 340 foods I analyzed, 255 contained added sugar. That amounts to over three fourths of the foods surveyed. You can confirm the accuracy of this by randomly selecting 20 items from the supermarket shelves and searching the labels for added sweeteners. At least half will contain sugar. The key is to recognize the names for the various forms of sugar as they are listed on the labels. In my survey corn syrup was the most frequent type followed by sugar (beet or cane) and dextrose. Other types of refined sugars commonly added to foods include invert syrup, malt syrup, maple syrup, refined honey, glucose, white grape juice concentrate, fructose, and fruit sugar concentrate. Refined vegetable oil, a category which includes margarine, hydrogenated oil, partially hydrogenated oil, lard, tallow, and liquid vegetable oil, was the second most common category listed. Nearly one half of all supermarket food contains such oils. MSG ran a close third. Other food additives which are found in a large percentage of grocery store items include:

white flour and rice	nitrates and other synthetic
corn starch	preservatives
synthetic iron	ethylene glycol
coal tar dyes	propylene glycol
yeast and yeast extracts	artificial flavors (derived)
sulfites	from petrochemicals)
refined milk products	caramel color

Hydrogenated Fats

Fats and oils are probably the most misunderstood, as well as maligned, of all foods. There is a general perception that if fats are derived from vegetables sources, they are health-enhancing, while animal fats are toxic. As a result, it has been assumed that vegetable oils, even those which are highly adulterated, are safer to consume than animal fats of any type, including yolk of egg, pure butter, cream, and the fat found naturally in meats.

Ironically, in terms of saturation, there is little difference between hydrogenated oils such as those found in margarine and the animal fats they are meant to replace, even though they are derived from vegetable sources. Here is why. Saturated fats are hydrogenated; that is the way they occur in Nature. This saturation explains why animal fats are hardened, that is they are solid at room temperature. In contrast, in Nature, vegetable oils are liquids, that is until they are hydrogenated by the oil manufacturers. Thus, in summary, the terms hydrogenation and saturation describe the condition of the oil molecule. If a fat molecule is saturated, it is solid at room temperature; if it is hydrogenated, it is also solid. In contrast, if it is unsaturated, it is in a liquid state at room temperature.

You may want to try an experiment, the results of which are rather shocking. Take an egg poaching pan; put butter into one of the egg cups and margarine in the other. Bring the water under the cups to a boil and note the time that each takes to melt. Hint: butter melts almost instantly, whereas margarine will not fully melt even after being subjected to the heat of boiling water for a full 10 minutes.

The consumption of hydrogenated oils has been linked with a variety of diseases, including heart disease, high blood pressure, hardening of the arteries, diabetes, multiple sclerosis, Alzheimer's disease, Parkinson's disease, arthritis, immune disorders, psoriasis, lupus, scleroderma, and cancer.

High cholesterol can result from eating margarine, contrary to the stance of the American Dietetic and American Heart Associations. In fact, recent studies published in prominent medical journals, such as the New England Journal of Medicine, document that margarine increases blood cholesterol levels to a greater degree than do natural cholesterol sources such as butter and eggs. The implication is obvious; always opt for the natural over the synthetic.

Do you consume on a daily, weekly, or monthly basis:

1. margarine
2. commercial peanut butter
3. non-dairy creamer
4. imitation whipping cream
5. microwave popcorn
6. Egg-Beaters
7. imitation ice cream
8. Wheat Thins, Triscuits, Ritz, Waverly Wafers, Cheez Nips, Bacon Thins, or similar snack crackers
9. cookies
10. doughnuts
11. Twinkies, cupcakes, Suzi-Q's, Ho-Hos, and/or similar snack cakes
12. fruit pies
13. cinnamon rolls and/or other sweet rolls
14. frozen or restaurant pizzas
15. fish sticks or other breaded fish pieces
16. Tater Tots
17. French fries
18. breaded tenderloins
19. breaded or batter-fried shrimp
20. breaded chicken
21. tortilla chips
22. Cheetos or cheese puffs
23. corn chips

24. potato chips
25. gelatin molds
26. cakes (homemade and/or commercial)
27. imitation cheese
28. burritos/tortillas
29. artichoke hearts in oil
30. scalloped potatoes
31. tacos
32. tartar sauce
33. kid-style commercial cereals (Trix, Lucky Charms, Cap'n Crunch, Cocoa Puffs, etc.)
34. hot chocolate
35. muffins, including bran muffins
36. brownies
37. pot pies
38. pancakes
39. waffles
40. fondue
41. "broiled" restaurant fish (or chicken)
42. chewy candies (jelly beans, Juji-Fruits, etc.)
43. Pop-Tarts
44. boxed soup mixes
45. creamed soups
46. creamed frozen vegetables
47. graham crackers
48. pretzels (some)
49. Archway-style "home-made" cookies
50. Oreo-style sandwich cookies
51. peanut butter cookies
52. chocolate chip cookies, fudge, or chocolate covered cookies
53. crescent rolls
54. doughnuts
55. cheese cakes
56. bread
57. hamburger/hot dog buns and/or dinner rolls

58. cheese popcorn
59. Velveeta-type cheese spread and/or Cheez Whiz
60. ice cream cakes or sandwiches
61. puddings and/or pudding pops
62. egg rolls
63. pasta-style frozen dinners
64. frozen hash browns

Your Score ____

1 to 15 points *Mild hydrogenated oil toxicity*: There truly is no such thing as mild hydrogenated oil toxicity, since any amount is toxic. These oils are not meant for human consumption. They cannot be found in Nature and are produced strictly as a result of the manipulation of the chemical structures of naturally occurring oils. Avoid all dietary sources of these oils. Strict avoidance is necessary, because hydrogenated oils, even in small amounts, can cause cellular damage via the mechanism of *lipid peroxidation*. The latter may be defined as the generation of rancid fats within human tissues. This may become manifested outwardly by aging of the skin as well as the deposition of unsightly brown spots, known also as *liver spots*. Certain nutrients, particularly vitamin E, beta carotene, bioflavonoids, pycnogenol glutathione, pantothenic acid, and selenium, help prevent lipid peroxidation.

16 to 29 points *Moderate hydrogenated oil toxicity:* You are consuming hydrogenated oils by the tablespoonful. Tissue damage will invariably occur if you continue consuming them. The cells of your body have no option but to attempt to utilize or absorb these distorted oils. As a result, the cell membranes become weakened or, more descriptively, they stiffen. This membrane damage leads to cellular malfunction, and, ultimately, disease may result. For instance, imagine a white blood cell possessing stiffened membranes; will it be

able to catch up with an invader? Stop eating all foods containing hydrogenated or partially hydrogenated oils and do not use margarine. Use butter instead. In addition, take the following supplements on a daily basis:

primrose oil - 8 capsules
vitamin E - 1200 I.U.
beta carotene - 50,000 I.U.
lecithin - 2 heaping tablespoons of granules
selenium - 600 mcg daily
ground flax - 3 heaping tablespoons daily
glutathione - 300 mg
vitamin C - 2,000 mg
pycnogenol - 90 mg

30 to 50 points *Severe hydrogenated oil toxicity*: You are consuming hydrogenated oils by the cupful. Carefully read all labels to ensure that absolutely no hydrogenated oils, partially hydrogenated oils, or margarine enter your diet.

The question may arise as to what should be done about the hydrogenated and partially hydrogenated oils already absorbed into the cellular membranes as a result of years and/or decades of consuming toxic/hydrogenated fats? Drive them out of the tissues with the essential fatty acids and their vitamin co-factors. Take the following supplements on a daily basis for at least two months:

primrose oil - 12 capsules
lecithin - 8 capsules
ground flax seed - 6 heaping tablespoonfuls (or two
tablespoons of pure cold-pressed flax seed oil)
B-6 and zinc - 50 mg of each (to aid in fatty acid
metabolism)
vitamin E - 1,600 I.U.
selenium - 600 mcg
N-acetyl cysteine - 1 gram

188

glutathione - 400 mg
pycnogenol - 180 mg

51 and above *Extreme hydrogenated oil toxicity*: You are consuming hydrogenated oils by the tubful. Eliminate all dietary sources of these oils immediately. Follow the afore-mentioned recommendations for nutritional supplements. However, increase the daily dosage of vitamin E to 2,000 I.U., pycnogenol to 300 mg and glutathione to 500 mg. Additionally, eat restaurant food with caution; it often contains added oils. Be sure to ask your server to have the chef cook your food *oil-free*. Butter and pure extra virgin olive oil may be acceptable alternatives if the recipe must call for oil. Even so, the restaurant environment is a difficult one to control for the diet-conscious individual, since only chefs can provide a definite answer to the question of whether refined vegetable oils, hydrogenated fats, or margarine are added to the food. What's more, it has recently been determined that some chefs start with pure olive oil but dilute it with refined oils such as cottonseed oil. This practice is reprehensible. Cottonseed oil is one of the least edible of all oils and is, in fact, not even a vegetable oil. It is a waste product of cotton harvesting and is sold for no other reason than to stretch the profit dollars reaped by the cotton industry. In other words, cottonseed oil is inedible. Furthermore, it is usually contaminated with significant amounts of pesticide and herbicide residues, more so than any other type of oil. Therefore, if you must use olive oil at a restaurant, ask the chef if he/she dilutes it with any other type of oil.

There is yet another problem in many restaurants: butter substitutes. Thousands of restaurants, under the guise of promoting good health, have switched from real butter to "Country Crock," "I Can't Believe It's Not Butter," "Promise," or similar butter/margarine substitutes. The servers often bring this vile mixture to the table whipped into a ball; it looks, smells, and tastes like butter. To make matters worse, if you ask the server what it is, he/she will tell you that *it is butter, pure butter, nothing added and nothing removed.* Waiters and waitresses simply cannot be relied upon to provide an accurate answer, since they truly believe that the butter substitute is real butter. What's more, restaurant employees are unaware that margarine is inferior to butter as a food source. Thus, it is your responsibility to demand that the server ask the chef (or go back to the kitchen and ask the chef yourself; I have done this on numerous occasions) to check labels in order to be certain that this "butter" is the real thing and is free of all additives, hydrogenated oils, and margarine. Only then can you be assured that you will be eating the real thing.

Deep Fried Food

There is a great deal of overlap between food containing hydrogenated oils and deep fried food. Every year, billions of pounds of hydrogenated oils, as well as liquid vegetable oils, are used for deep frying food, both in restaurants and at home. These oils are also used in baking as well as in the manufacture of a wide range of packaged food. The distinction between this and the previous exam is that the deep fried food listed herein may be defined as food cooked in a deep fryer, wok, pot, or skillet, resulting in the saturation of the food with additional refined vegetable oil, lard, and/or tallow.

When dining at home or in restaurants, do you consume on a daily, weekly, or monthly basis:

1. French fries, home fries, and/or American fries
2. fried shrimp
3. fried chicken

4. onion rings
5. fried vegetable sticks and/or mushrooms
6. cheese balls
7. fried fish
8. corn dogs
9. chicken fried steak
10. chicken Kiev
11. breaded chicken breasts and/or chicken nuggets
12. Chinese food entrees
13. won tons and egg rolls
14. egg fu yung
15. stir fry
16. potato skins
17. omelets (not cooked in butter)
18. fried hot fruit pies and/or ice cream
19. hot Vienna beef and/or sausage (deep fried)
20. fondue
21. doughnuts
22. Hush-Puppies
23. tenderloins

Your Score _____

1 to 5 points *Mild deep fried oil toxicity:* Eating any amount of deep fried oils is too much. These oils are heated to incredibly high temperatures, plus they are used repeatedly. Essentially, these oils are cooked and re-cooked until they turn black, a process which astronomically increases their toxicity. Deep fried oils are poisonous; avoid them entirely. In addition, take 800 I.U. of vitamin E daily to protect your body from rancid oil-induced toxicity.

6 to 13 points *Moderate deep fried oil toxicity:* You are consuming dangerously high amounts of deep fried oils. The foods you are eating are coated and infiltrated with them. Cellular damage is assuredly occurring. Eating refined and

hydrogenated vegetable oils increases the risks for cancer, heart disease, multiple sclerosis, Alzheimer's disease, Parkinson's disease, lupus, diabetes, psoriasis, and arthritis. These oils provoke inflammation and depress immunity. Eliminate all dietary sources of refined vegetable and deep frying oils and stop eating deep fried food at restaurants.

Refined vegetable oils destroy vitamin E, and, thus, individuals who consume large amounts of deep fried food are deficient in this nutrient. To correct this deficiency, take a minimum of 1200 I.U. of vitamin E daily. Additionally, take daily dosages of the following antioxidants: vitamin C (2,000 mg), glutathione (300 mg), and beta carotene (25,000 I.U.).

14 and above *Severe deep fried oil toxicity:* You are consuming deep fried oils by the cupful. Stop eating these noxious oils immediately. It is likely that you are suffering from a sort of addiction to deep fried food, a propensity which I call *The Hot Grease Syndrome.* The toxicity and tissue damage caused by these oils can be reversed by consuming large amounts of antioxidants and by permanently avoiding the consumption of deep fried food. Take the following supplements on a daily basis in divided dosages for at least two months:

    vitamin E - 2,000 I.U.
    organic selenium - 500 mcg
    vitamin C - 3,000 mg
    beta carotene - 100,000 I.U.
    glutathione - 400 mg
    aged garlic extract (Kyolic) - 9 capsules daily

In addition, take essential fatty acids: 6 tablespoons of ground flax seed and 12 capsules of primrose oil on a daily basis.

The White Flour Quiz

White flour is found in thousands of supermarket foods. It is a subtle food additive. In other words, it is so easy to disguise that people are usually unaware that they are eating it. For example, are you aware that it is a primary component of creamed soups, including most of those served in restaurants? It is listed on food labels in various forms, including flour, white flour, wheat flour, bread crumbs, wheat starch, malt, and maltodextrin. What all of these forms have in common is the fact that they contribute unnecessary calories, while providing no flavor and minimal nutritional value.

All commercial white flour contains inorganic iron, which is added to the flour during the fortification process. The refinement and bleaching of flour destroys approximately 70% of its vitamin content and as much as 90% of its mineral content. Nearly 30 nutrients are depleted and/or destroyed during the refining of crude whole wheat kernels into white flour. The only nutrients which are returned are thiamine, riboflavin, niacin, and vitamin B-6 as well as the iron. Thus, white flour and the foods made from it, such as pasta and noodles, cannot be deemed nutritious in any respect.

White flour should be avoided for another reason: it is devoid of fiber. Because of this, it causes bowel disorders, particularly colitis, diverticulitis, and constipation. If you must eat flour, consume whole grains. Better yet, purchase a whole-grain food processor and grind your own flour from fresh grain kernels. Such "farm-fresh" whole grains offer the following benefits, as contrasted to the whole grain products available in the supermarket:

1) They are free of toxicity; most whole grains are rancid by the time you purchase them.
2) They are richer in vitamins and minerals than commercial pre-ground whole grains.

3) They are easier to digest and far less likely to provoke allergic reactions.
4) They taste better.

Do you consume on a daily, weekly, or monthly basis:

1. crackers
2. pretzels
3. loaf bread
4. hot dog and/or hamburger buns
5. corn bread and/or Hush Puppies
6. rolls
7. Twinkies, Zingers, Cup-Cakes, Little Debs, and similar dessert cakes
8. doughnuts
9. cookies
10. chow mein noodles
11. canned soups
12. creamed vegetables
13. breaded chicken
14. breaded seafood
15. bread dressing
16. gravies
17. pizza
18. egg rolls
19. croutons
20. pasta-style TV dinners
21. spaghetti
22. lasagna
23. macaroni and cheese
24. canned macaroni dishes (Spaghettios, ravioli, etc.)
25. French toast
26. waffles
27. pancakes
28. crepes
29. ice cream pies, cakes, or sandwiches

30. ice cream cones or drumsticks
31. cakes (commercial or home-made)
32. pot pies
33. burritos/tortillas
34. bagels
35. creamed soups
36. commercial cereals (cold)
37. commercial hot cereals containing wheat (Malt-o-Meal, Cream of Wheat, etc.)
38. malted milk and/or Ovaltine
39. muffins, including bran muffins
40. Pop-Tarts
41. broth soups with noodles
42. chunky soups
43. graham crackers
44. saltines
45. dumplings
46. croissants
47. tea or fruit cakes
48. breaded tenderloins
49. fruit pies
50. sweet rolls, including cinnamon rolls
51. candy bars containing cookies or wafers
52. pudding
53. batter breads (date-nut, pumpkin, banana, etc.)
54. flat or unleavened breads (pita, matzo, etc.)

Your Score ____

1 to 12 points	*Mild white flour overload*
13 to 23 points	*Moderate white flour overload*
24 to 34 points	*Extensive white flour overload*
35 and above	*Massive white flour overload*

At all levels of overload it is advisable to reduce white flour intake. Foods containing white flour are poor food choices. Ideally, bleached white flour should never be consumed.

Replace white flour products with unprocessed whole grains such as coarse whole wheat, oat meal, grits, whole rye, crude corn meal, brown rice, and wild rice. Alternative grains or grain-like foods include amaranth, teff, quinoa, spelt, kamut, and buckwheat. These may be purchased in health food stores and are less likely to provoke allergy reactions than the more common grains.

White flour is inedible, because it is devoid of nutrients. Its fiber is stripped away, its vitamins are destroyed by refining and bleaching, and its minerals are almost entirely removed. Those who score in the extensive or massive category have an additional concern: inorganic iron toxicity. That is because all white flour and white flour products are fortified with iron as iron sulfate, a chemical form little different from iron filings. When ingested over a prolonged period, inorganic iron may cause liver damage and may also increase the risk for heart disease and cancer.

Some of the most valuable scientific studies on iron toxicity in humans were performed by Richard G. Stevens, PhD. His monumental research, which was published in the *American Journal of Clinical Nutrition*, documented as much as a threefold increased risk for these diseases depending upon the degree of elevation in the iron levels. These figures apply only to men and post-menopausal women, both of whom have low nutritional requirements for iron. Since it is difficult to eliminate via the normal excretory pathways, iron readily accumulates within the tissues. Thus, men and post-menopausal women should curtail the consumption of grains fortified with inorganic iron, and that means all foods containing white flour and rice, including pasta.

White flour is pure starch. This starch consists molecularly of sugar molecules attached by chemical bonds. Once ingested, the starch of white flour is rapidly broken down into glucose. In sedentary individuals the glucose is poorly utilized and is usually converted into triglycerides or fat. Thus, the consumption of white flour products is a contributing factor in the cause of blood sugar disturbances, obesity, high triglycerides, and high cholesterol as well as heart disease itself.

The Pasta Quiz

Pasta has been touted as a health food particularly over the last 20 years. Currently, it is hailed as the ideal replacement for traditional dishes, such as meat, fish, and poultry, primarily because of its low fat content.

There is a certain degree of overlap between this exam and the previous one, since pasta is made from white flour. Yet, it serves to emphasize a point; commercial pasta is nothing more than white flour molded into a variety of shapes. It is no more health enhancing than eating white bread and is one of the major sources for the ingestion of inorganic iron in the American diet.

Do you consume on a daily or weekly basis:

1. soup with noodles, pasta shells, or "alphabets"
2. spaghetti
3. pasta dishes and/or entrees in restaurants
4. hamburger helper and/or similar products
5. salads containing pasta
6. Spaghettios or goulash
7. ravioli
8. macaroni and cheese
9. pasta-style TV dinners
10. lasagna

Your Score _____

Any score means you are consuming an excess of pasta. Pasta offers no significant nutritional value in terms of vitamins and minerals. In addition, it contains inorganic iron, which destroys vitamins A, C, E, and K.

Spinach, soy, and whole wheat pasta provide a wider range of nutrients than the standard commercial types. However, the difference is not significant; vitamins and minerals are found scattered in commercial grain flours in trace amounts. If the objective is to consume nutrient-dense foods, pasta is a poor choice. For as many calories as it contains and as much poundage as it can put on, superior food selections can be made in the quest to eat nutritionally.

No doubt, Americans love eating grains. In fact, millions of Americans are addicted to grains, this being largely the result of food allergy. Even so, whole grains, if fresh and properly prepared, are relatively good sources of vitamins and minerals and are loaded with fiber. You don't have to give up whole grains forever; just eat them judiciously.

Refined Milk Products

Pure unprocessed milk is a wholesome food, just as is whole wheat. However, like wheat, milk can be refined to such a degree that its nutritional value is disrupted or destroyed. The primary concern in milk adulteration is homogenization, a process which alters the natural chemistry of the milk. Homogenization breaks milk's naturally large fat globules into microscopically tiny globules. These globules are absorbed directly into the bloodstream and fail to undergo the natural digestive processes necessary to render them nontoxic. While unprocessed whole milk, despite its fat content, is a safe food, evidence exists that the consumption of large quantities of homogenized milk may contribute to heart disease.

Skim and non-fat dry milk are the primary types of refined milk products used as food additives. Other refined milk derivatives commonly found in processed foods include calcium caseinate (or casein), milk solids, whey, butter solids, and caramel coloring.

Do you consume on a daily or weekly basis:

1. reduced fat ice cream
2. ice milk (swirl cones, Dairy Queen, etc.)
3. puddings and/or custards
4. coffee creamers
5. non-fat dry milk
6. evaporated or condensed milk
7. skim or one percent milk
8. Cheetos, Cheez Nips, cheese popcorn, or similar snacks
9. skim milk (hard) cheeses
10. low-fat cottage cheese
11. fudgesickles, froststicks, Bon Bons, Drumsticks, Eskimo Pies, Dove bars, or similar products
12. artificial cream or eggs
13. artificial ice cream
14. Velveeta, Cheez Whiz, and/or similar processed cheese products
15. processed American cheese
16. hot chocolate
17. creamed vegetables
18. creamed soups
19. gravies
20. cookies (some)
21. yogurt (non-fat or low-fat)
22. artificial sour cream
23. processed cheese dip
24. nachos or cheese tortilla chips
25. caramels and/or taffy
26. chocolate coated candy bars and/or chocolates
27. Do you drink 3 or more glasses of milk daily?
28. Do you consume foods containing caramel coloring?

Your Score _____

The advice for all of these categories is the same: avoid processed milk products and/or foods containing them. As an alternative select fresh milk products made from whole milk. Use cream instead of coffee creamer. If you must drink milk, drink pure whole milk instead of skim or 1% milk. However, it is advisable to keep the milk consumption at one glass or less daily, unless you have access to certified non-homogenized milk. If you are sensitive to milk, use goat's milk, which is easier to digest and less allergenic than cow's milk.

Certain individuals are intolerant to all types of milk. Many of these individuals suffer from a condition known as *lactose intolerance.* Rather than being an allergy, this condition is due to a deficiency of the enzyme required for breaking lactose (i.e. milk sugar) into its component parts. The unabsorbed lactose irritates the intestines, causing bloating, cramps, indigestion, and/or diarrhea. Lactose intolerance can be corrected simply by taking capsules of the missing enzyme, *lactase*, whenever consuming milk products. However, allergy to milk products is extremely common in the United States. Thus, even fresh whole milk products are unacceptable food sources for certain individuals.[12]

---

12. Chemical contamination of commercial milk is another concern. Dairy cattle are routinely administered antibiotics and hormones, residues of which are commonly found in milk. Of perhaps greater concern is the FDA's approval of bovine growth hormone (BGH) for use in stimulating milk production. The safety of this hormone is dubious. Certain evidence links its use to growth disturbances in children as well as tumor development.

The Yeast-in-Foods Quiz

Yeasts are added to foods for several reasons. They are leavening agents. They are also added to enhance flavor. Additionally, they are sources of nutrients, notably B-complex vitamins and protein.

Virtually all baked goods contain yeast, and this is particularly true of breads, buns, muffins, rolls, cakes, and doughnuts. The rule of thumb is that if it is raised and/or has a crust, it contains yeast. A variety of terms are used for describing yeast additives on food labels, including:

autolyzed yeast protein
hydrolyzed vegetable protein
vegetable protein
baker's yeast
brewer's and torula yeast

Fermented foods and beverages are another major source of yeasts. This is because yeasts are commonly used as starters for fermented foods, or they may multiply within the foods as a result of the fermentation process. Such foods and beverages include baked goods, alcoholic beverages (particularly wine and beer), vinegar, soy sauce, and cheese.

Yeasts are toxic only to people who are sensitive to them. Allergy to yeasts may result in a variety of symptoms, including rashes, vaginitis, colitis, asthma, intestinal gas, bloating, indigestion, cold/flu syndromes, sinusitis, painful joints, and migraine headaches.

Do you consume on a daily, weekly, or monthly basis:

1. bagels
2. crackers
3. cookies
4. pretzels

201

5. pancakes and/or waffles
6. cracker crumbs and/or croutons
7. dry roasted nuts (some)
8. breaded foods
9. canned soups (some)
10. TV dinners
11. bologna
12. breakfast strips
13. ravioli
14. noodles and/or lasagna
15. pizza
16. Sloppy Joe mix
17. broth soups and/or bouillon
18. protein powders
19. boxed soup mixes
20. breads (including pita bread)
21. hamburger and/or hot dog buns
22. dinner rolls, muffins and/or croissants
23. soy sauce (some)
24. egg rolls
25. sweet rolls, cake, and/or doughnuts
26. pasta-style TV dinners
27. breaded fish and seafood
28. aged cheeses
29. horseradish
30. pot pies
31. root beer
32. vitamin tablets containing yeast
33. alcoholic beverages, particularly beers and wines
34. vinegar
35. batter cakes (date-nut, pumpkin, banana, etc.)

Your Score _____

1 to 9 points   *Mild dietary yeast overload*
10 to 19 points   *Moderate dietary yeast overload*
20 to 28 points   *Severe dietary yeast overload*
29 and above   *Extreme dietary yeast overload*

For each of these categories the advice is the same: reduce the consumption of foods containing yeast. This is particularly true for individuals who have a history of multiple food allergies. Such individuals are often allergic to dietary yeasts and may suffer violent reactions upon ingesting foods containing them. Thus, those who suffer from allergy-induced diseases, such as candidiasis, hives, bronchitis, asthma, arthritis, colitis, eczema, sinusitis, mental illness, ear infections, and migraine headaches, are likely to benefit greatly from a yeast-free diet. In particular, asthmatics who score high on this exam (above 20) are likely to achieve a rapid improvement if dietary sources of yeasts are thoroughly eliminated.

Inorganic Iron Quiz

This quiz covers essentially the same material as the white flour and pasta quizzes. However, it is included to emphasize a point; many Americans are unknowingly consuming vast amounts of inorganic iron. Since iron is one of the few nutrients which steadily accumulates in the body and since it is potentially toxic, it is important that people know where they stand in terms of iron intake.

For every 10% increase in tissue iron stores above normal the risk for certain diseases, notably heart disease, arthritis, and cancer, is nearly doubled. Thus, in many individuals the intake of inorganic iron should be restricted just as the consumption of MSG, sulfites, sugar, and caffeine should be eliminated or reduced. Men, as well as post-menopausal women with normal blood counts, should significantly reduce their consumption of foods fortified with inorganic iron and should never take supplements containing it. Such individuals usually receive all the iron they need from consuming foods naturally rich in this nutrient such as red meats, eggs, and spinach.

Medically, iron toxicity is known by the terms *hemosiderosis* and *hemochromatosis*. The distinction between these two conditions is primarily the fact that the latter is a more serious illness, involving a greater degree of iron deposition within critical internal organs. Both are associated with toxic accumulations of iron in a wide range of tissues, including the skin, mucous membranes, liver, spleen, lymph glands, pancreas, joints, pituitary, and heart.

Hemosiderosis and hemochromatosis are difficult to diagnose based upon clinical presentation alone. That is because the symptoms are often vague and are commonly observed in a variety of other conditions. However, by combining symptom evaluation with a thorough blood analysis, the diagnosis can be readily determined. Symptoms of iron toxicity include weakness, severe fatigue, loss of appetite, abdominal pain, chronic infection, diarrhea, nausea, and weight loss. In addition, iron toxicity may initially present with the classic symptoms of diabetes: weight loss, fatigue, excessive thirst, and frequent urination. This is due to the fact that the excessive iron causes destruction of the pancreas, specifically those cells responsible for the synthesis of insulin.

Excessive iron accumulation may not be due exclusively to increased iron intake. It may be the result of a genetic defect in iron metabolism/absorption. Individuals with the defective gene absorb iron at an accelerated rate, as much as ten times normal. Researchers have discovered that iron absorption can be blocked by consuming megadoses of certain minerals such as calcium, magnesium, silicon, and zinc.

The existence of iron overload can be confirmed by blood testing. If you scored high on this exam, be sure to see your doctor and request that the appropriate tests be performed. Only then can you be certain that iron toxicity exists.

Do you consume on a daily or weekly basis:

1. pasta
2. bread (pita, leavened, unleavened)
3. hot dog and/or hamburger buns
4. dinner rolls and/or croissants
5. creamed vegetables
6. muffins
7. bagels
8. sweet rolls and/or doughnuts
9. burritos and tortillas
10. cupcakes, Twinkies, Suzi Qs, or similar desserts
11. red meats (a rich source of organic iron)
12. cookies
13. cakes and/or pies
14. waffles and/or pancakes
15. Pop-Tarts
16. pretzels
17. creamed soups
18. commercial cereals (most)
19. Malt-O-Meal, Cream of Wheat, and/or similar hot cereals containing wheat
20. malted milk
21. croutons
22. brownies
23. boxed or canned soups with noodles
24. multiple-vitamins containing iron
25. Have you received numerous blood transfusions (8 or more)?
26. Do you have a history of an elevated red blood cell count (polycythemia or leukemia)?
27. Do you drink red wines on a daily or weekly basis?
28. Do you cook in an iron skillet often?

29. Do you take iron pills or Geritol even though you are not anemic?

Your Score ____

1 to 7 points *Mild iron toxicity:* Inorganic iron, even in relatively small amounts, may provoke tissue damage. Men don't need the extra iron. Avoid all foods fortified with iron. Vitamins containing iron should also be avoided. Iron-free multiple vitamins are available at many health food stores, or call Nutritional Supplement Service, 800-243-5242.

9 to 15 points *Moderate iron toxicity:* At this level of iron overload tissue damage is likely to occur. Further accumulation may significantly increase the risks for degenerative diseases such as diabetes, arthritis, lupus, multiple sclerosis, hardening of the arteries, heart disease, and cancer. Follow the previously mentioned advice, being particularly careful to avoid all iron-fortified foods. Take an iron-free multiple mineral tablet as an aid to blocking iron absorption. Increase the consumption of calcium-rich foods, since this mineral is the most effective one for preventing iron absorption.

16 to 22 points *Severe iron toxicity:* Adhere to the previously mentioned advice, being sure to carefully check all food labels for added iron. In addition, strictly avoid alcohol consumption, since it markedly increases iron absorption. Blood tests for iron overload are indicated. Supplement the diet on a daily basis with a multiple-mineral (iron-free) in addition to 1,000 mg of calcium.

23 and above *Extreme iron toxicity:* Warning—at this level of iron intake the risks for a variety of degenerative diseases, including cancer, arthritis, heart disease, lung disease, Alzheimer's disease, lupus, diabetes, multiple sclerosis, and liver disease, are greatly increased. Follow the previously

mentioned advice, strictly avoiding all dietary sources of iron. In addition, take the following minerals on a daily basis: calcium (2,000 mg), zinc (60 mg), magnesium (1,000 mg), and silica (2,000 mg).

In extreme cases of iron overload food sources of iron, such as red meats, spinach, red wine, prunes, and raisins, must also be reduced or eliminated. See your doctor and request blood tests for iron overload, including serum iron and ferritin levels. If the ferritin level is excessively high (above 200), therapeutic phlebotomy may be necessary. Levels above 350 may be an early signal of internal malignancy.

The Refined Sugar Quiz

The majority of commercial foods available in America are laced with refined sugars. These sugars, which include white sugar, corn syrup, glucose, dextrose, and fructose, are the most commonly used of all food additives. In fact, they are so commonly found in food that the consumption of refined sugars in America exceeds 120 pounds per person per year. That is an incredibly large amount of sugar to be ingesting. Just imagine; it amounts to every American woman, man, or child eating a ten-pound bag of pure sugar every month.

Refined sugars are found in an inordinate number of commercial foods. Regardless of their forms or names, all refined sugars react within the body in a similar manner, resulting in the predictable nutritional and health defects which refined sugar is known to cause. The dilemma is that the sugar offers no nutritional value, being devoid of all traces of vitamins, minerals, enzymes, and proteins. In fact, this hidden sugar is creating a wide range of health problems; both physical and mental symptoms often occur as a result of the consumption of disguised sugar. Of perhaps greater concern is the rising incidence of diseases directly related to sugar consumption: diabetes, stroke, cancer, senility, arthritis, hypertension, schizophrenia, and heart disease. What's more, many of these diseases are developing at an alarming frequency in children and adolescents. Almost everyone knows a child who suffers from high cholesterol or an adolescent plagued by juvenile diabetes. Scientific studies have correlated the consumption of refined sugar with the rising incidence of heart disease, high cholesterol, behavioral disorders, learning deficit, blood sugar disorders, obesity, and diabetes in children as well as adolescents and adults. Does it make sense to perpetuate this problem by continually feeding the youth sugar-infested foods?

In many respects adults, particularly the elderly, exhibit an even greater vulnerability to the noxious effects of refined sugar than do children. Sugar increases cholesterol and triglyceride counts, damages arterial linings, heightens blood pressure, irritates the kidneys, disrupts adrenal function, depresses immunity, and agitates the nervous system. Elderly individuals frequently develop mental impairment as a result of excessive sugar intake. Parkinsonism, Alzheimer's disease, chronic depression, psychotic behavior, and senility have all been correlated with sugar overload. The fact is sugar consumption plays a greater role in the cause of these diseases than the substances typically associated with their genesis such as aluminum, iron, lead, pesticides, etc. A number of symptoms commonly experienced by the elderly, such as poor attention span, memory loss, insomnia, anxiety, agitation, irritability, confusion, hostility, fatigue, cold extremities, pruritus, and weakness, are provoked or caused by the ingestion of refined sugar. Thus, all individuals would feel better, think more clearly, and probably live longer if they curbed or curtailed their sugar intake.

As mentioned previously, the average American consumption of refined sugar is over 120 pounds per person per year. Yet, this is only the average. It means that some individuals consume 200 or perhaps 300 pounds of sugar per year. Think about it. That's two or three ten-pound bags of sugar per month. Few people would knowingly consume that much sugar. The problem is that Americans have grown accustomed to eating food products liberally laced with a variety of refined sugars. Sugar has been added to disguise the fact that the nutrients and naturally occurring flavors have been processed out. Plus, it makes the food addictive.

Do you consume on a daily, weekly, or monthly basis:

1. Hershey's, Cadbury, or other milk chocolate bars
2. Snickers, 3-Musketeers, Mars Bars, or Milky Ways
3. Nestle's Crunch or Mr. Goodbars
4. salted nut rolls
5. Butterfingers or Baby Ruths
6. (other) candy bars
7. chocolates, Hershey's kisses, or chocolate bark
8. ketchup
9. sweet relish and/or pickles
10. corn relish
11. canned sweet corn
12. pickled beets
13. cup cakes
14. brownies
15. fudge
16. sugar-sweetened cereals
17. cured luncheon meats
18. ice cream or ice milk
19. malts or shakes
20. sherbet
21. after-dinner mints
22. non-dairy creamer
23. whipping cream (artificial or canned)
24. taffy, caramels, and/or Milk Duds

25. applesauce
26. pudding
27. canned fruit in heavy or light syrup
28. honey-roasted nuts
29. homemade salad dressings sweetened with sugar
30. jelly beans
31. Juji Fruits or similar chewy treats
32. peanut butter cups
33. Zingers, Twinkies, and/or Suzi-Qs
34. oatmeal pies
35. caramel corn
36. taffy apples
37. flavored yogurt
38. vanilla wafers
39. M & M type candies
40. canned soups
41. pretzels
42. boxed soup mixes
43. graham crackers
44. Wheat and/or Oat Thins
45. jellies and jams
46. refined honey
47. apple butter
48. commercial peanut butter
49. crescent rolls
50. marshmallows and marshmallow cream
51. Pringle's-style potato chips
52. bread
53. hamburger and hot-dog buns
54. caramel corn, Poppy Cock, and/or Cracker Jacks
55. hot dogs
56. ham
57. bacon and/or breakfast strips
58. turkey and/or chicken salad
59. bean dip
60. Jello and/or gelatin molds

61. pickled herring
62. sausage links and/or summer sausage
63. bean and/or potato salad
64. marinara (pasta) sauce
65. canned yams
66. pickled red cabbage
67. hash browns and/or Tater Tots
68. canned chili
69. Spaghettios
70. bagels
71. Sloppy Joe mix
72. steak sauce and/or taco sauce
73. barbecue sauce and/or barbecued meats
74. commercial salad dressings (mayonnaise)
75. French, Roquefort, Western, thousand island, blue cheese, ranch, and Caesar dressings
76. pancake mixes
77. frozen or prepared waffles or pancakes
78. sno-cones and/or slushes
79. Buster Bars, Dilly Bars, fudgesickles, drumsticks, or ice cream sandwiches?
80. pudding pops
81. Bomb Pops, Mr. Freeze pops, and popsickles
82. cookies
83. gum sweetened with sugar
84. hard candies
85. doughnuts
86. pies
87. pastries
88. peanut brittle
89. fruit salad
90. pecan rolls
91. Tootsie Pops and/or other suckers
92. Tootsie Rolls

93. mousses
94. baklava or similar exotic ethnic sweets
95. chutney/bottled seasonings
96. peanut clusters
97. peppermint and/or lemon drops
98. yogurt-coated nuts/candies
99. rootbeer floats and/or chocolate sodas
100. chocolate covered raisins, nuts, malted milk balls, etc.
101. Whip 'n Chill type deserts

Your Score ____

1 to 18 points *Mild refined sugar toxicity:* While this level of intake is listed as mild, it is still significant. It would be preferable to satisfy the desire for sweets with fresh fruits, pure raw honey, sweet vegetables, or juices. These at least contain some valuable nutrients. Be sure to take a B-complex supplement and a multiple-vitamin/mineral tablet containing chromium. This will aid in the effort to break the sugar habit by reducing cravings.

19 to 34 points *Moderate refined sugar toxicity:* If you suffer from fatigue, irritability, PMS, headaches, allergies, sinus problems, memory loss, irregular heartbeat, frequent colds/flu, fungal infections, itchy skin, sleep disorders, mood swings, and/or depression, sugar is the likely culprit. Refined sugar is addictive. Resolve the sugar addiction immediately before further tissue damage occurs. To aid you in this battle, take megadoses of B-vitamins and chromium, which are required to process/digest sugar and help reduce sugar cravings. Try also megadoses of tyrosine (2 grams), co-enzyme Q-10 (100 mg), and pantothenic acid (2 grams); all of these nutrients boost the adrenal glands' anti-sugar response.

35 to 65 points *Severe refined sugar toxicity:* You are consuming refined sugar by the handful each day. Curtail this excessive sugar intake immediately. Follow the previously mentioned advice and take 200 to 300 mcg of chromium several times daily. Additionally, take magnesium (1 gram), potassium (300 mg), selenium (300 mcg), manganese (15 mg), and silica (500 mg), since sugar induces deficiencies of all of these nutrients. Try megadoses of pantothenic acid, 1500 mg three or four times daily. If the cravings persist, add 1 gram of glutamine three times daily. Do whatever it takes to lick the sugar habit.

66 and above *Extreme refined sugar toxicity:* You are consuming refined sugar by the bowlful each day (or each week). As a result your internal organs literally are becoming corroded. The greatest damage is being inflicted upon the liver, colon, pancreas, adrenal glands, thyroid gland, and pituitary gland. Stop this destructive sugar addiction immediately. Take the following nutritional supplements:

B-complex - one or two tablet(s) three times daily
chromium - 500 mcg three times daily
manganese - 4 mg three times daily
tyrosine - 1000 mg three times daily
pantothenic acid - 2000 mg three times daily
glutathione - 1 gram three times daily
coenzyme Q-10 - 100 mg three times daily
rice polishings - 3 tablespoons three times daily
glutamine - 1 gram three times daily
selenium - 300 mcg daily

Stay on these supplements for at least 90 days after you break the sugar habit. Then reduce the dosage by 50% as a maintenance.

The Refined Sugar in Beverages Quiz

Here is an astounding statistic: Americans consume a greater volume of fluid as soft drinks than water. If beer were included as a soft drink (it is more hard than soft), water would be a major loser.

Everyone knows that soft drinks are a primary source of sugar in the American diet. In fact, these drinks constitute fully 25% of all sugar consumption. The sugar in these drinks is readily disguised by a variety of coloring agents (including caramel) if not subtly by the colorful graphics of the soft drink containers. It is odd that people drink soft drinks without considering that all they are getting nutritionally is pure sugar. These same individuals might think twice about drinking the homemade equivalent of a typical cola: seven to eight teaspoons of white sugar stirred into a twelve ounce glass of carbonated water. Yet, it is not just soft drinks that are major sources of "drinkable" sugar. There are literally hundreds of other drinks containing sugar, many of which are listed as follows:

Do you consume on a daily or weekly basis:

1. Kool Aid
2. colas (including Dr. Pepper)
3. Hi-C and/or fruit punch
4. grape, lemon, lime, or orange juice drink
5. chocolate milk
6. hot chocolate (or hot cocoa)
7. coffee or tea with sugar
8. coffee or tea with coffee creamer
9. Ovaltine, PDQ, or Nestle's Quick
10. instant breakfast
11. Slim-Fast or similar weight loss drinks
12. lemonade

13. malted milk
14. malts and shakes
15. ice cream sodas
16. ice slushes
17. sweetened ice tea
18. "health drinks" sweetened with grape sugar, apple juice, or corn syrup
19. refined apple juice
20. peach, pear, apricot, or guava nectar
21. cranberry juice cocktail
22. liqueurs
23. mixed drinks containing added sugar
24. Gatorade and/or similar athletic drinks
25. Ensure and/or similar supplemental drinks
26. Tang
27. 7-Up, Sprite, or Mountain Dew
28. root beer
29. fruit flavored sodas (Orange Crush, grape soda, etc.)
30. Do you drink 2 or more cans/bottles of pop every day? (If so, add 5 points to your total)

Your Score _____

1 to 5 points	*Mild sugary drink toxicity*
6 to 12 points	*Moderate sugary drink toxicity*
13 to 19 points	*Severe sugary drink toxicity*
20 and above	*Extreme sugary drink toxicity*

For all categories the treatment is the same; stop consuming drinks containing sugar, corn syrup, caffeine, and food dyes. Drink instead beverages that are health-enhancing such as pure fruit and vegetable juices, unsweetened protein shakes (such as *Nutri-Sense*), and water. Individuals who score on the high end of the severe or extreme category have an increased risk for certain illnesses, notably low blood sugar, diabetes, tooth decay, pyorrhea, anxiety, depression, lupus,

PMS, endometriosis, and heart disease. Additionally, excessive intake of sugar greatly impairs the immune response, predisposing individuals to a wide range of infectious conditions, including colds, flu, pneumonia, bronchitis, ear infections, and, particularly, yeast infections. This is largely because sugar destroys selenium, zinc, vitamin C, pantothenic acid, and pyridoxine, all of which are necessary for maintenance of normal immunity.

Food Dye Quiz

Food processors are convinced that foods must be adulterated with artificial colors in order to make them appear more appetizing. Thus, they add all manner of food colorings to enhance visual appeal and stimulate purchasing. No consideration is given regarding the food value or potential toxicity of these dyes. Rather, the only concern is "what will sell." Thus, thousands of foods contain synthetic dyes made from coal tar and petrochemical residues, these dyes being descriptively known as *artificial colors*.

I observed an interesting event illustrating the effects of food dyes on living tissues. I was in the wilderness—fishing in Canada. One of our party was far from nutritionally oriented; he brought along a couple of quarts of Gatorade. This drink consists largely of refined sugar and food dyes. We caught and cleaned fish from the pristine waters of the Canadian wilderness—pure white fillets of walleyed pike. The fish were placed in the refrigerator with the intent of preparing them later for supper. When I removed them, the flesh of the fish had turned pink—the Gatorade, since it was placed on its side in the small refrigerator, had leaked into the fish container. The red dye had leached into the fish, essentially "pickling them" irreparably, and no amount of washing could salvage them. I explained to my companion that this was precisely what was happening to his internal organs when he consumed Gatorade or similar drinks laced with food dyes. Only time will tell whether my use of logic will have any positive effect on this individual's dietary habits.

The FDA keeps tabs on food dyes by issuing numbers for each of them. You can tell if a food dye is synthetic and, therefore, toxic in two ways: if the label lists the terminology "artificial color(s)" or if it is listed as a numbered dye such as FD&C #5. All of these dyes are documented carcinogens. My philosophy is no level is safe. Carefully read all labels and avoid foods containing artificial dyes. Certainly do not add food dyes to your foods. It is possible to have a happy Easter without coating eggs with toxic food dyes.

Do you consume on a daily, weekly, or monthly basis:

1. pickles
2. relish
3. dinner rolls (some)
4. popsickles
5. Kool-Aid
6. gelatin
7. hard candies
8. chewing gum (or bubble gum)
9. Gatorade
10. sno cones and slushes
11. fruit drinks and/or punch
12. puddings
13. pie fillings
14. frostings
15. artificial cheese and processed sliced cheeses
16. canned fruit
17. colored cereals
18. marshmallows (colored or white)
19. sherbet
20. Mountain Dew
21. apple and cherry turnovers

22. wine coolers
23. commercial multiple vitamins
24. coated or colored drugs
25. red, orange, yellow, blue, or green colored candies
26. birthday and/or layer cakes
27. fruit, upside down, and tea cakes
28. imitation cheese
29. maraschino cherries and/or crab apples
30. frozen pizzas
31. microwave popcorn
32. Trix, Lucky Charms, Fruit Loops, and similar colored cereals
33. thousand island dressing
34. ice cream (especially fruit-flavored)
35. canned frosting
36. orange, yellow, or green colored pop
37. Cool Whip or similar imitation whipped toppings
38. grape or orange drink (including Hi-C)
39. Pop Tarts
40. pudding pops
41. margarine
42. crescent rolls (and also some hot-dog/hamburger buns)
43. doughnuts
44. sweet rolls
45. cheese cake

Your Score _____

1 to 8 points *Mild food dye toxicity:* Food dyes are toxic even in minute quantities. These chemicals are proven carcinogens. Avoid them as you would avoid the plague; do not feed your children food dye-contaminated foods.

9 to 18 points *Moderate food dye toxicity:* You are consuming excessive amounts of processed foods contaminated with food dyes. Change your diet by eating wholesome,

unprocessed foods instead of devitalized, chemically poisoned junk foods.

19 to 30 points *Severe food dye toxicity:* At this level of intake a variety of symptoms are likely to occur, including depression, headaches, agitation, joint pain, fatigue, sinus problems, cold/flu, and irritability. In children, food dyes may cause or provoke a variety of mental illnesses such as attention deficit disorder, behavioral defects, delayed learning, depression, autism, and even seizures.

Asthmatics are particularly vulnerable to the toxic effects of food dyes and may exhibit severe allergic reactions. In fact, thousands of fatal and near fatal reactions have resulted from the ingestion of food dyes. The main culprit is Yellow Dye #5. Also known as tartrazine, this coal tar derivative is the asthmatic's processed food nightmare. The chemical belongs to the aspirin family. Thus, aspirin-sensitive asthmatics, of which there are millions, are exceptionally sensitive to it. Asthmatics must scrutinize the labels of all processed foods for such terms as food dyes, artificial colorings, artificial flavorings, tartrazine, and Yellow Dye #5.

31 and above *Extreme food dye toxicity:* Warning—the consumption of large amounts of food dyes over prolonged periods increases the risks for a variety of cancers. Follow the previously mentioned advice, being sure to carefully eliminate all dietary sources of these carcinogens. Individuals suffering from chronic disease who registered in the extreme category will invariably notice an improvement after eliminating dietary sources of synthetic dyes.

It is essential that you regard this advice seriously and alter your diet immediately. If you are an asthmatic, removing food dyes from the diet may be a matter of life and death.

MSG Quiz

MSG, or monosodium glutamate, is a synthetic chemical which is commonly added to processed foods. It is described on some food labels as a "flavor enhancer." Not surprisingly, it is devoid of nutritional value. In fact, it may be toxic even in relatively small quantities.

Dr. George Schwartz's book, *In Bad Taste: The MSG Syndrome*, classifies MSG as a drug-like substance. Further, he claims that "MSG is a poison...," which would not be surprising, since drugs produce their actions by poisoning cellular functions. To illustrate the widespread occurrence of MSG in foods, Dr. Schwartz notes that MSG is found in *"most of the food* prepared by major fast-food chains (italics mine)." Moreover, he notes that as many as 20 million Americans, or nearly one-tenth of the population, are known MSG reactors. He proposes that in all probability this figure could be tripled to include those who are unknowingly sensitive to it. This latter figure is supported by laboratory data. Studies on MSG toxicity describe a consistent picture; nearly one-third of animals and humans tested reacted negatively in some fashion after ingesting MSG. What's more, certain subjects developed intense and potentially dangerous symptoms. The researchers concluded that, in highly sensitive individuals, permanent disability may result from toxic MSG reactions.

MSG is truly a hidden food additive. Usually, it can't be seen, touched, smelled, or even tasted. To make matters worse, it is often disguised on food labels under names besides MSG. Schwartz notes that the term MSG is less commonly found on food labels than the toxin's disguised names: hydrolyzed vegetable protein, autolyzed yeast, modified food starch, and "natural" flavors. Thousands of processed foods have these terms listed on their labels, and all are taboo for those who are MSG-sensitive.

Do you consume:

1. fish sticks or patties
2. tortilla chips
3. potato chips
4. Cheetos or cheese puffs
5. soy sauce
6. canned stew
7. processed cheese
8. Planters dry roasted nuts (other brands also may contain MSG)
9. croutons and bread crumbs
10. canned tuna (Chicken of the Sea, Geisha, Bumble Bee, or S&W)
11. canned chunky beef, chicken, or turkey
12. canned chicken, ham, turkey, or beef spread
13. canned Chinese foods
14. canned ravioli, Beefaroni, or spaghetti and meatballs
15. pizza (especially frozen types)
16. egg rolls
17. breaded chicken (i.e. fried chicken, chicken nuggets, etc.)
18. TV dinners
19. breaded shrimp, clams, and/or scallops
20. submarine sandwiches
21. pepperoni
22. hot dogs and/or corn dogs
23. bologna and/or salami
24. pastrami
25. tenderloins
26. breakfast strips
27. egg substitutes
28. baked beans
29. creamed vegetables
30. scalloped and/or au gratin potatoes
31. tomato sauce (some)

32. chili
33. prepared sliced turkey, beef, or chicken (deli-style)
34. Sloppy Joe mix
35. pudding
36. taco sauce
37. ketchup
38. tartar sauce (some)
39. mayonnaise
40. thousand island dressing
41. French, ranch, or Caesar dressing
42. chicken-fried, Salisbury, or Swiss steak
43. beef Stroganoff
44. artificial ice cream
45. frozen waffles
46. cream soups
47. broth soups and/or canned soup broth
48. steaks, chops, or poultry seasoned with Accent or Lawry's seasoning
49. Oriental restaurant food
50. boxed soup mixes
51. chunky soups
52. doughnuts, sweet rolls and/or cupcakes
53. fruit pies
54. cup cakes
55. bean dip
56. cheese dip (some)
57. peanut butter cookies (some)
58. flavored yogurt (some)

Your Score ____

1 to 10 points *Mild MSG toxicity:* If you are an MSG reactor, even tiny amounts must be avoided. This is particularly true if you suffer from allergy-induced illnesses such as arthritis, hyperactivity, attention deficit disorder, asthma, hives, obesity, or migraines.

11 to 22 points *Moderate MSG toxicity:* You are consuming a significant amount of MSG on a daily or weekly basis. It is likely that the MSG is accumulating in your tissues and causing toxicity. This can result in a variety of mental symptoms and may ultimately contribute to the cause of certain diseases. Curtail the consumption of MSG and MSG-tainted foods. The following nutrients may be useful in reducing MSG toxicity:

    vitamin C - 1,000 mg twice daily
    vitamin E - 1200 I.U. daily
    selenium - 400 mcg daily
    beta carotene - 25,000 I.U. daily
    fat-soluble thiamine - 200 mg daily
    B-complex - 1 tablet twice daily

23 to 41 points *Severe MSG toxicity:* You are consuming large amounts of MSG on a daily basis. Migraine headaches, flu-like symptoms, sinusitis, memory loss, depression, agitation, and anxiety are common MSG-induced syndromes. The consumption of this compound is probably responsible for many of your ailments. In all likelihood you are addicted to MSG, and the reactions it causes in your body may be turning you into a nervous wreck. Go cold turkey and remove all dietary sources of MSG. Take the following nutritional supplements to aid in preventing withdrawal symptoms and to heal any toxic damage that may have developed within the nervous system:

    vitamin C - 1,000 mg three times daily
    vitamin E - 1200 I.U. daily
    selenium - 300 mcg twice daily
    beta carotene - 50,000 I.U. daily
    fat-soluble thiamine - 400 mg daily

tyrosine - 1 gram twice daily
B-complex - 1 tablet three times daily
magnesium - 400 mg twice daily
choline - 2 grams daily
B-6 - 50 mg daily

42 and above *Extreme MSG toxicity:* Warning—neurological damage may occur as a result of prolonged consumption of large amounts of MSG. At this level of intake MSG-induced imbalances in brain chemistry are virtually assured. Severe depression, agitation, and even suicidal ideation may result. To help reverse MSG-induced damage and neurological imbalances, as well as to aid in curing the addiction, take the following brain chemistry enhancing agents:

tyrosine - 1 gram three times daily
niacin - 100 mg three times daily
B-complex - 2 tablets three times daily
B-6 - 50 mg twice daily
folic acid - 5 mg twice daily
magnesium - 400 mg twice daily
calcium - 500 mg three times daily
fat-soluble thiamine - 200 mg three times daily

In addition, take the following antioxidants in order to heal the nervous system damage/toxicity:

vitamin C - 2,000 mg three times daily
vitamin E - 800 I.U. twice daily
selenium - 250 mcg three times daily
beta carotene - 25,000 I.U. twice daily
glutathione - 200 mg twice daily
essential fatty acids - 9 capsules daily

Sulfites Quiz

Sulfites are a class of chemicals derived from the gaseous compound sulfur dioxide. The toxicity of sulfur dioxide is well known. This is the compound responsible for acid rain.

Sulfites and sulfur dioxide are added to foods in order to preserve their appearance. Sulfites offer no nutritional value and, in fact, destroy nutrients, notably vitamin C, vitamin A, vitamin E, vitamin B-12, riboflavin, and molybdenum. Asthmatics are particularly vulnerable to reacting to the toxicity of sulfites, and several deaths have occurred as a result of sulfite allergy.

Dozens of symptoms result from sulfite reactions. These symptoms include rashes (particularly hives), sinus congestion or runny nose, sinus pressure, headaches, achiness, cold sweats, diarrhea, joint pain, chest pain, shortness of breath, swelling of the face, throat, tongue, or lips, and sudden bouts of fatigue. Sulfites are unfit for human consumption.

Do you consume:

1. cole slaw
2. dried fruits
3. white and brown sugar
4. potato salad
5. pies
6. hard candy
7. gelatin (Jello)
8. fruit drinks
9. fruit salad (fresh, frozen, or canned)
10. frozen vegetables
11. guacamole
12. tortilla chips
13. canned soups
14. deli fruit or salads

15. fruit toppings and fillings
16. jams and jellies
17. pancake mixes
18. pancake syrup
19. cornstarch
20. instant tea
21. hard liquor
22. breakfast drinks
23. gravies and sauces
24. salad dressings
25. TV dinners
26. French fries, Tater Tots, or American fries
27. hash browns
28. horseradish (some)
29. frozen fruit (some)
30. sauerkraut
31. scalloped or au gratin potatoes
32. instant mashed potatoes
33. soy sauce (some)
34. vinegar (most)
35. fruit pies
36. wine and wine coolers
37. restaurant foods cooked in wine

Your Score _____

1 to 9 points *Mild sulfite toxicity:* Even at this low level of intake highly sensitive individuals might exhibit toxicity. Usually, such individuals have a history of allergy manifested by asthmatic attacks, allergic rashes, hives, sinus problems, and/or migraine headaches. Individuals who exhibit sensitivity must avoid all dietary sources of sulfites.

10 to 19 points *Moderate sulfite toxicity:* Sulfites are poisonous and, once ingested, are converted to the highly toxic gas, sulfur dioxide. Sulfites and their metabolites

suppress immunity and provoke allergic reactions. Curtail the consumption of all food containing sulfites and take the following nutrients in order to detoxify the residues of this poison:

- vitamin B-12 - 500 mcg daily
- folic acid - 1 mg daily
- vitamin C - 1,000 mg twice daily
- molybdenum - 100 mcg twice daily
- methyl sulfonyl methane (MSM) - 100 mg twice daily

20 to 28 points *Severe sulfite toxicity:* Warning—serious injury and/or death may occur in highly sensitive individuals as a result of the consumption of large amounts of sulfites. Allergic reactions to sulfites include hives, rashes, sinus disturbances, headaches, shortness of breath, and sore throats. Avoid all dietary sources of sulfites and take the following supplements:

- vitamin B-12 - 1,000 mcg daily
- folic acid - 2 mg twice daily
- vitamin C - 1,000 mg three times daily
- molybdenum - 50 mcg three times daily
- selenium - 200 mcg twice daily
- methyl sulfonyl methane (MSM) - 150 mg twice daily

29 and above *Extreme sulfite toxicity:* You are consuming massive amounts of the highly oxidative sulfites on a daily basis. If you have a significant history of allergy and/or asthma, your life may be at risk. Sulfite-induced asthmatic attacks, throat edema, and shock are serious reactions; dozens of deaths have resulted from such toxic insults. Immediately curtail the intake of all dietary sources of sulfites. Always ask the preparers/servers at restaurants if sulfites are added to

the food. In addition, take the following sulfite antagonists and detoxifying agents:

- vitamin B-12 - 1,000 mcg three times daily
- folic acid - 2 mg three times daily
- vitamin C - 2,000 mg three times daily
- vitamin A - 25,000 I.U. twice daily
- molybdenum - 200 mcg three times daily
- organic selenium - 200 mcg twice daily
- N-acetyl cysteine - 100 mg twice daily
- methyl sulfonyl methane (MSM) - 200 mg three times daily

The Nitrated Meats Quiz

Nitrates are added to meats as preservatives primarily to prevent microbial growth. However, they also are utilized to improve visual appeal, since they turn the meat a brighter color, giving it a reddish tint. Excessive dietary intake of nitrates is linked to heart disease, diabetes, stroke, and cancer.

The cancer-causing effects of nitrates have been thoroughly investigated. When nitrates or nitrites are ingested, they are converted in the stomach and intestines to compounds of even greater toxicity called *nitrosamines*. The toxicity of nitrosamines is so profound that they are regarded as one of the most potent of all known carcinogens. Nitrosamines damage the lining of the stomach and intestines by destroying cellular genetic material. Chronic consumption of nitrates with their subsequent formation into nitrosamines significantly increases the risks for stomach, intestinal, esophageal, bladder, and liver cancer.

The transformation of nitrates to nitrosamines is blocked by certain foods, vitamins and minerals. Researchers discovered that nitrosamine formation within the intestines is prevented if the diet is rich in vitamin C. Other nutrients which inactivate nitrosamines and/or prevent their formation include beta carotene, glutathione, selenium, bioflavonoids, riboflavin, and vitamin E. Aged garlic extract is even more powerful than these nutrients. Recent research conducted in Asia determined that garlic extract (Kyolic was the brand used) was ten times more effective than vitamin C in inactivating nitrosamines.

Cigarette smoke is another major source of nitrosamines. Every puff initiates a chain reaction leading to nitrosamine formation within the tissues, particularly the lungs, liver, and digestive tract. In fact, according to the internationally renowned cancer researcher Kedar Prasad, author of *Vitamins Against Cancer*, cigarette smoke is the number one environmental source of nitrosamines. This largely accounts for the powerful cancer-causing actions of tobacco smoke.

Tap water is an additional significant source of nitrates. The major source of nitrates in water is agricultural run-off of nitrogenous fertilizers and animal wastes. When ingested these nitrates can also be converted to nitrosamines.

Do you consume:

1. pork and beans
2. ham
3. salami and/or summer sausage
4. bologna
5. head cheese and/or pickled pigs feet
6. bacon and/or breakfast strips
7. corned beef and/or corned beef hash
8. pastrami
9. hot dogs and/or corn dogs
10. smoked turkey breast
11. Spam
12. sausage
13. turkey salami, bologna, or ham

14. beef jerky
15. chipped beef
16. bratwurst
17. liverwurst
18. pepperoni and/or Canadian bacon
19. Do you eat smoked fish (including lox)?
20. Do you eat fresh fruits and vegetables only rarely?
21. Do you live in an area of heavy air pollution?
22. Do you smoke cigarettes on a daily basis? *(Note:* if you smoked 2 packs or more for longer than five years, add an additional 5 points to the final score)
23. Are you exposed to passive smoke on a daily basis?
24. Do you smoke pipes or cigars?
25. Do you use chewing tobacco?
26. Do you drink tap water derived from water tables in an area of heavy agriculture?

Your Score _____

1 to 6 points *Mild nitrate toxicity:* Nitrosamines are potent carcinogens. Thus, no amount of dietary intake of nitrates can be deemed safe. Since nitrates and particularly nitrites are readily converted to nitrosamines, the consumption of nitrated meats should be restricted or preferably curtailed. Be sure to take Japanese aged garlic (Kyolic) extract as well as extra amounts of vitamin C (at least 2,000 mg per day) to help clear the noxious nitrates out of the system.

7 to 12 points *Moderate nitrate toxicity:* At this level of intake the risks for cancer and heart disease rise significantly. Eliminate all dietary sources of nitrates, including smoked foods. Avoid barbecued meats. Protect yourself from unavoidable secondhand smoke and pollution by taking large doses of antioxidants, particularly vitamin E, beta carotene, vitamin A, vitamin C, selenium, and glutathione. Take Kyolic aged garlic extract, 9 capsules daily.

13 to 18 points *Severe nitrate toxicity:* Warning—the amount of nitrates you are consuming greatly increases your risks for heart disease and cancer. Stop the intake of all nitrated and smoked meats. If you are a smoker, quit immediately. If you are exposed to significant amounts of second hand smoke, do whatever is necessary to protect yourself, e.g. make your spouse smoke outside the house, etc. The consumption of large doses of antioxidants and other nutrients which prevent or reverse nitrate-induced toxicity will help stimulate the healing of damaged tissues. Take the following nutrients on a daily basis for at least two months:

- organic selenium - 600 mcg
- beta carotene - 100,000 I.U.
- vitamin C - 4,000 mg
- vitamin E - 1600 I.U.
- glutathione - 300 mg
- zinc - 50 mg
- pantothenic acid - 2,000 mg
- vitamin B-6 - 50 mg
- folic acid - 5 mg
- aged garlic extract - 12 capsules daily

19 and above *Extreme nitrate toxicity:* You are consuming nitrates and nitrites by the teaspoonful. Nitrosamine formation is assuredly occurring in your internal organs. The risk for developing life-threatening diseases, particularly cancer, heart disease, and diabetes, is exceedingly high. If you are a migraine headache, arthritis, or asthma sufferer, it is likely that dietary nitrates are contributing to the cause. If you are a smoker, your life is at risk unless you quit immediately. Stop consuming nitrated meats and/or other sources of nitrates, before it is too late. Follow the supplemental program listed previously; however, increase the dosage of vitamin C to 6,000 mg, glutathione to 500 mg, and vitamin E to 2000 I.U.

The Caffeine and Caffeine-Like Substance Quiz

Caffeine can be descriptively called the "nervousness" food additive. It is one of the most powerful of all addictive substances, and millions of Americans are knowingly or unknowingly habituated. However, caffeine addicts don't take it simply to get wound up. Rather, they consume caffeine because it gives them a jolt of energy, albeit temporary. Since the energy they receive is artificial, caffeine addicts continually "reach for the pot" to maintain their sensation of nervous energy.

Caffeine is technically listed as a drug and is, in fact, an ingredient in dozens of over-the-counter as well as prescription medications. Yet, it is freely added to foods in amounts which produce drug-like effects.

This test evaluates the consumption of food/beverage sources of caffeine, as well as caffeine-like substances, the latter being found primarily in cocoa- and vanilla-flavored foods. Both cocoa and vanilla beans contain nervous system stimulants from the same chemical family as caffeine. These stimulants are known collectively as *methylxanthines*.

Caffeine is a neurotoxin. If consumed continually, it readily accumulates within the tissues, since it takes approximately eight hours to fully metabolize. What's more, it tends to preferentially accumulate within the tissues of the nervous system: the brain, spinal cord, and peripheral nerves. Thus, with repeated daily doses of caffeine, it is possible to develop caffeine toxicity. This is especially true for those suffering from liver or kidney disease, since these organs are involved in the excretion and detoxification of caffeine. In other words, if the function of these organs is impaired, toxic amounts of caffeine rapidly accumulate in the tissues.

Do you consume on a daily or weekly basis:

1. caffeinated coffee
2. iced tea
3. black or green tea
4. herbal teas containing black tea
5. colas containing caffeine
6. Mountain Dew
7. chocolates or chocolate-coated candy bars
8. chocolate milk
9. cookies containing chocolate chips
10. chocolate malts, shakes, and/or sodas
11. chocolate covered ice cream bars
12. coffee flavored candy and/or ice cream
13. cookies flavored with cocoa or vanilla bean extract
14. chocolate or vanilla flavored cake
15. ice cream flavored with cocoa or vanilla bean extract
16. candy bars containing vanilla bean extract
17. chocolate or vanilla pudding
18. chocolate mousse or Whip 'n Chill
19. brownies or fudge
20. almond bark
21. cappuccino
22. hot chocolate
23. Dr. Pepper
24. Are you currently taking theophylline (asthma medication)?
25. Do you have a history of endometriosis and/or fibrocystic breast disease?
26. Do you consume drugs which contain caffeine (e.g. Excedrin, Caffergot, etc.)?
27. Do you have a history of kidney and/or liver disease?
28. Do your hands tremble after consuming caffeinated substances?
29. Do you become nervous, moody, and/or agitated after consuming caffeinated substances?

30. Do you develop a headache, or do you become irritable if you fail to get your caffeine fix?
31. Do you binge on and/or crave chocolate?
32. Do you drink 6 or more cups of coffee per day? (if so, add an additional 5 points to your final score)

Your Score _____

1 to 6 points *Mild Caffeine Toxicity:* For some individuals caffeine is toxic in any amount. This may be partially the result of an allergy-like sensitivity to the substance. If you are caffeine-sensitive or if you have a history of PMS, endometriosis, migraine headaches, ulcerative colitis, or fibrocystic breast disease, avoid even small amounts of caffeine and caffeine-like substances.

7 to 15 points *Moderate Caffeine Toxicity:* You are consuming excessive amounts of caffeine and caffeine-like substances on a daily or weekly basis. As a result, a variety of symptoms are probably occurring, including insomnia, agitation, nervousness, mood swings, breast tenderness, PMS, migraines, colitis, tremors, and headaches. If you have symptoms of caffeine-induced illness, curtail the consumption of all dietary sources of caffeine, cocoa, and vanilla bean. In addition, take the following supplements in order to detoxify the residual caffeine:

- pantothenic acid - 1,000 mg twice daily
- vitamin C - 500 mg twice daily
- selenium - 200 mcg twice daily
- tyrosine - 500 mg twice daily
- choline - 500 mg twice daily
- vitamin B-6 - 25 mg twice daily

16 to 23 points *Severe Caffeine Toxicity:* The caffeine you are consuming is causing toxicity within your nervous system. Immediately stop the intake of dietary sources of caffeine. However, due to the risk of withdrawal reactions, go cold turkey only after beginning the following nutritional supplement program:

- pantothenic acid - 1,000 mg twice daily
- vitamin C - 1,000 mg twice daily
- folic acid - 1 mg twice daily
- B-complex - 1 tab twice daily
- tyrosine - 1,000 mg twice daily
- vitamin B-6 - 50 mg twice daily
- choline - 500 mg twice daily
- inositol - 500 mg twice daily
- rice polishings - 2 heaping tbsp. twice daily

24 and above *Extreme Caffeine Toxicity:* Warning—caffeine and/or coffee, if consumed in massive amounts, may cause genetic damage. Studies document that heavy coffee consumption results in damage to genetic material, which has been determined by detecting the existence of abnormal chromosomes in the urine. In addition, the risk for pancreatic cancer is significantly increased for those who consume in excess of five cups of coffee per day. Curtail your excessive caffeine/coffee consumption immediately. Be aware of the side effects of going cold turkey: depression, agitation, anxiety, nervousness, shaking/tremors, anger, frustration, insomnia, digestive disturbances, constipation, fatigue, and headaches. To help control or minimize these symptoms, initiate the following nutritional supplement program prior to discontinuing the caffeine:

- folic acid - 1 mg three times daily
- B-complex - 1 tab three times daily
- tyrosine - 1,000 mg three or four times daily
- choline - 1 gram twice daily
- inositol - 1 gram twice daily
- fat-soluble thiamine - 300 mg twice daily
- selenium - 300 mcg twice daily
- rice polishings - 2 heaping tbsp. twice daily

Section III

Illnesses and Syndromes

The "Are You Aging?" Quiz

No one wants to become old. Yet, everyone ultimately comes, figuratively speaking, "face to face" with this concern. While each of us will become older, we do not have to look excessively old. It is not inevitable to lose teeth, develop failing eyesight, suffer hearing loss, become bald and/or gray, or shrivel up like a prune. Rather, aging can be blocked, delayed, or controlled. Thus, it is possible to retain a certain degree of vitality and vigor, as well as a youthful appearance, despite reaching old age. A "feel and act young" attitude is essential, but so is an adequate supply of the nutrients which stall the aging process. This is because aging occurs primarily from the inside out and the essential nutrients decrease the rate of aging that occurs within vital internal organs.

Certain nutrients have been studied extensively for their anti-aging properties. These nutrients exert their effects whether taken internally or applied externally. In fact, the combination of external and internal application of anti-aging nutrition is one of the secrets to maintaining one's beauty and physique well into old age. As only one example of the value of nutrients in reversing aging, researchers recently (1992) reported that taking vitamin C supplements on a regular basis may extend lifespan by as much as six years. Just think what could be accomplished in aging delay if a broad spectrum of anti-aging nutrients were consumed on a regular basis.

Certain dietary factors accelerate the aging process. Excessive eating is one of them. The per capita caloric consumption in America is astronomically high and is nearly twice that of primitive societies. Researchers are thoroughly documenting the fact that fasting or moderate food abstinence helps retard the aging process and may extend lifespan by as much as ten years.

The skin is a barometer of how rapidly an individual is aging. Americans often marvel at how elderly individuals from non-Western societies appear young and how their skin remains beautiful. These individuals follow a diet closer to an "all-natural" one which is relatively free of the toxic substances replete in the American diet. These toxic substances may be descriptively called *aging factors*. They include refined vegetable oils, hydrogenated oils, refined sugar, inorganic iron, nitrates, synthetic food additives, caffeine, and cigarette smoke (separate exams are found within this book for each of these items).

There are a number of external as well as internal signs which give evidence that accelerated aging is occurring. Some of these signs may have triggered your concern already. Take this quiz to see how rapidly you are aging.

Which of these apply to you?

1. crow's feet (lines radiating from the eyes)
2. bags under the eyes
3. loss in the elasticity of the skin
4. noticeable thinning of the skin
5. cholesterol deposits on the face and/or eyelids
6. raised brown or flesh-colored spots on the face or hands
7. moles that are increasing in number and/or changing in appearance
8. age spots (liver spots) on the face, hands, or arms
9. vitiligo (white spots due to a loss of pigment on the skin)
10. wrinkle lines on the face radiating from the upper lip toward the nose
11. excessive wrinkling of the face, arms, chest, and/or hands
12. receding gums
13. deepening wrinkle lines on the forehead
14. tiny red capillary spots on the face, arms, chest, or legs
15. a noticeable tilting forward of the head and neck

16. nodular growths on the face, nose, hands, or chest
17. loose skin or bags under chin and/or arms
18. stiffening of the spine
19. generalized decrease in joint mobility
20. pain and/or deformity of the joints
21. reduction of the size of the upper lip
22. tendency to shuffle instead of stride while walking
23. ridges on the fingernails
24. increasing occurrence of varicose and/or spider veins
25. gradual (or sudden) decline in visual capacity
26. constant coldness of the hands, feet, arms, legs, face, and/or ears
27. skin that is easily damaged by sunlight
28. dryness of the mucous membranes (nose, vagina, sinuses, mouth, etc.)
29. generalized dryness of the skin
30. one bowel movement or less per day
31. circular lines around the skin of the neck
32. receding hairline or balding (or, in women, massive hair loss)
33. graying of the hair
34. skin tags
35. dryness of the eyes and/or nasal passages
36. persistent tremors
37. heart arrhythmia (irregular heartbeat)
38. rapid heartbeat (80 or more beats per minute)
39. floaters in the eyes
40. loss of muscle tissue in the arms, shoulders, and/or legs
41. Have you noticed a reduction in the size of fingers and/or wrists (i.e. reduced ring size)?
42. Are you becoming increasingly fatigued as the years go on?
43. Are you currently a heavy smoker (one-half pack or more per day)?
44. Have you previously smoked one-half pack or more per day for a period longer than five years?

45. Do you or did you live in the same house as a heavy smoker (who smokes in the house)?
46. Are you currently a heavy drinker (six or more drinks per week)?
47. Had you previously been a heavy drinker for more than five years (six or more drinks per week)?
48. Do you or did you consume large amounts of cane sugar or other refined sugars added to foods or as hidden food additives on a daily or weekly basis?
49. Do you or did you eat deep fried foods, such as French fries, fried chicken, fried fish, etc., on a daily or weekly basis?
50. Do you or did you regularly consume nitrated and/or preserved meats (hot dogs, ham, bacon, pastrami, bologna, corned beef, salami, jerky, etc.)?
51. Do you currently work or have you in the past worked closely with volatile petrochemicals (e.g. gas station attendants, furniture refinishers, refinery workers, glue workers, road tarring crews, etc.)?
52. Are you exposed to excessive amounts of sunlight without protection (proper clothing, sunscreen)?
53. Are your teeth cracking or chipping?
54. Are you suffering from an increasing degree of muscular weakness?
55. Do you suffer from hearing loss?
56. Do you have a total or near total loss of taste or smell?
57. Do you suffer from macular degeneration, retinopathy, or retinal detachment?
58. Do you suffer from loss of peripheral vision?
59. Are you becoming increasingly vulnerable to injuries (sprains, strains, bruises, cuts, etc.)?
60. Is your hair becoming fine or thin, or is it dull in appearance?
61. Is your recovery time becoming increasingly delayed after becoming ill with colds, flu, or other infections?

62. Do you have a history of heart disease, stroke, and/or hardening of the arteries?
63. Have you been diagnosed with internal cancer?
64. Have you been diagnosed with skin cancer?
65. Have you been diagnosed with osteoporosis?
66. Do you have a history of cataracts?
67. Do you have high blood pressure?
68. Do you have psoriasis and/or eczema?
69. Do you use prescription drugs on a daily basis? (If you take 4 or more drugs, add an additional 5 points.)

Your Score ____

1 to 16 points *Minimal aging:* The key to preventing further aging is to follow a twofold approach: improve the diet and take the basic antioxidants as an insurance program to retard the aging process. This should include 2,000 mg of vitamin C, 1200 I.U. of vitamin E, 400 mcg of selenium, 25,000 I.U. of beta carotene, and 1,000 mg of pantothenic acid. Additionally, take an iron-free multiple vitamin, a B-complex tablet, and 60 mg of pycnogenol. The latter is a potent antioxidant extracted from the bark of pine trees. Avoid refined foods such as sugar, white flour, white rice, and commercial vegetable oils.

17 to 29 points *Moderate aging:* Take the antioxidants as described, increasing the daily dosage of beta carotene to 50,000 I.U. and the pycnogenol to 90 mg. In addition, take supplemental antioxidant enzymes, particularly glutathione (300 mg), coenzyme Q-10, riboflavin, and superoxide dismutase (SOD). Reduce your intake of refined sugar, and if you are a smoker, quit before it is too late. Eliminate from the diet all sources of refined vegetable oils. Avoid all nitrated and smoked meats. Curtail or reduce your consumption of alcohol. Apply an anti-aging skin cream to your hands and face on a daily basis.

30 to 42 points *Severe aging:* In addition to the previously mentioned dietary and supplemental advice, take 200 mg of coenzyme Q-10 each day. As aging becomes severe, tissue levels of coenzyme Q-10 decline dramatically. Increase the beta carotene dosage to 70,000 I.U., the vitamin C dosage to 4,000 mg, and the vitamin E dosage to 1800 I.U. Take 3,000 mg of pantothenic acid daily. If you are developing large numbers of brown, age, or liver spots, take 240 mg of pycnogenol daily, a potent antioxidant extracted from the bark of pine trees. Consume large amounts of the anti-aging vegetables, a category which includes turnips, radishes, carrots, beets, dark greens, cabbage, broccoli, kale, kohlrabi, onions, artichokes, watercress, and garlic. Apply an anti-aging cream to the face and hands morning and night.

43 and above *Extreme aging:* Warning—aging is occurring at a highly accelerated rate both externally and internally. In order to block or reverse this trend, take exceptionally high doses of anti-aging nutrients. In addition, protect your skin from further aging by applying topically the anti-aging nutrients. Supplement your diet with daily doses of the following nutrients:

- vitamin C - 6,000 mg
- vitamin E - 2200 I.U.
- beta carotene - 120,000 I.U.
- thiamine - 100 mg
- riboflavin - 100 mg
- pyridoxine - 100 mg
- pantothenic acid - 4000 mg
- PABA - 3,000 mg
- organic selenium - 600 mcg
- manganese - 6 mg
- chromium - 600 mcg
- silica - 3,000 mg
- calcium - 1500 mg

- magnesium - 800 mg
- potassium - 300 mg
- coenzyme Q-10 - 300 mg
- glutathione (or N-acetyl cysteine) - 500 mg
- pycnogenol - 300 mg

The last item on this list, pycnogenol, is one of the most potent antioxidants known and is some 20 to 50 times more powerful than vitamins C and E (for availability see Appendix C). Additionally, daily consume antioxidant enzymes, including glutathione reductase, catalase, peroxidase, and superoxide dismutase. Certain herbs and spices, such as garlic, oregano, cumin, coriander, fenugreek, and turmeric, possess properties which impede aging. Raw nuts and seeds, particularly almonds, sesame seeds, and sunflower seeds, possess substances which decelerate aging. Load up on foods and spices which block the aging process. Anti-aging fruits include strawberries, cherries, kiwis, papayas, mangoes, and grapefruits. Try the Anti-Aging Vegetable Juice Cocktail (see Appendix B). Apply an anti-aging cream to exposed skin morning and night (see Appendix C).

It is crucial that you alter your diet, since poor dietary habits are the major factor contributing to aging. Processed foods must be replaced by wholesome foods such as fresh fruits, vegetables, nuts, seeds, whole grains, and organic meats. Strictly avoid substances which accelerate aging. These substances include refined sugar, white flour, commercial vegetable and deep-frying oils, alcohol, toxic chemicals (and their fumes), chewing tobacco, and cigarette smoke. If you smoke, stop immediately. If you are exposed to secondhand smoke, make the changes necessary to prevent exposure.

Fasting is also advised, since food abstinence significantly deters the aging process. However, individuals suffering from serious medical conditions must undergo fasts only while under a physician's care.

The Sluggish Thyroid Syndrome

The Sluggish Thyroid Syndrome is perhaps the most commonly occurring hormonal disturbance in America today. It afflicts millions of people of all ages and sexes, although adult women are its usual victims. The thyroid gland controls the metabolic rate and is descriptively known as the "master of metabolism." As many as one in four Americans suffer from reduced thyroid function. Reduced body temperature is perhaps the most common consequence of impaired thyroid function. The individual who wears several extra layers of clothes, wears socks to bed, or who has "ice cold hands" is typically thyroid deficient.

As the master of metabolism, the thyroid gland exerts control of several critical functions, including body temperature, digestive enzyme synthesis, stomach acid production, fuel combustion, fat and protein synthesis, white blood cell synthesis and activity, and blood flow. The thyroid gland is also a critical player in the synthesis and activity of sex hormones.

Thyroid disorders are particularly common in the region of North America known as the *goiter belt*. This region was so named because of the high incidence of goiter that occurred there early in this century. This is essentially a pathological enlargement of the thyroid gland. Scientists determined that the states/provinces of the goiter belt had very low iodine levels in their soil and drinking water. Thus, the local food supply was lacking in this critical trace element, and unless an individual regularly consumed seafood, derangement of thyroid function and/or goiter was virtually assured. This "epidemic" was essentially obliterated via the introduction of iodized salt. Even so, goiter, as well as the related condition of thyroid nodules, remains a significant cause of illness in the goiter belt, which includes Ohio, Michigan, Indiana, Illinois, Wisconsin, Ontario, and Manitoba.

Which of these apply to you?

1. lethargy or weakness
2. tired in the morning and energetic at night
3. dry or coarse hair and/or skin
4. slow or slurred speech
5. swelling of the face and/or eyelids
6. cold hands and feet
7. bloating and indigestion after eating
8. hair loss from the outer third of the eyebrows
9. short-term memory loss
10. depression which is worse in the winter or on overcast days
11. white spots on the fingernails
12. chronic weight problems
13. easily constipated
14. PMS and/or other menstrual difficulties
15. infertility
16. swelling of hands and/or ankles
17. chronic headaches
18. emotionally unstable
19. brittle nails or nails which grow slowly
20. lack of sweating
21. poor appetite and/or lack of hunger
22. hair loss from the scalp, legs, and/or arms
23. generally nervous
24. difficulty getting deep breaths
25. heart palpitations
26. severe muscle cramps, especially at night
27. tendency to bruise easily
28. joint stiffness
29. require prolonged periods to get "warmed up" after exposure to cold
30. excessive appetite (never get full)
31. slow growing hair and/or nails
32. light or heavy menstrual flow

33. brittle hair
34. cholesterol deposits on the face or eyelids
35. lack of sexual desire
36. enlarged facial pores
37. poor hand-to-eye coordination
38. hoarseness or coarse voice
39. inability to translate thoughts into action
40. Do you tend to become depressed in the winter or after exposure to the cold?
41. Do you have a history of ovarian cysts?
42. Do you have repeated breast inflammation and/or infections?
43. Have your periods stopped prematurely?
44. Have you been diagnosed with low stomach acid (hypochlorhydria)?
45. Do you fail to feel rested even after sleeping long hours?
46. Do you have heart disease or hardening of the arteries?
47. Do you have cystic breast disease (lumpy breasts)?
48. Have you noticed that your skin has developed a yellowish tint?
49. Do you have chronic migraine headaches manifested by pain over the bridge of the nose, along the temple, or behind the eyes?
50. Do you drink fluoridated water and/or use fluoridated toothpaste?
51. Do you receive regular fluoride treatments from your dentist, or do you administer them at home?
52. Do you have high cholesterol and/or triglyceride levels?
53. Do you suffer from cracks in the bottom of the heels?
54. Are you morbidly obese and/or do you have a difficult time losing weight?
55. Do you have a history of repeated miscarriages?
56. Do you have a history of carpal tunnel syndrome?
57. Do you smoke a half pack or more of cigarettes per day?

58. Are you constantly cold even if you wear extra layers of warm clothing?
59. Do you have a low body temperature?

Your Score _____

1 to 11 points *Mildly sluggish thyroid:* Slight imbalances in thyroid function are common and usually can be corrected through dietary means. However, it may be necessary to supplement the diet with thyroid-boosting nutrients such as zinc, copper, magnesium, potassium, tyrosine, B-vitamins, iodine, and vitamin C. Take a multiple vitamin/mineral containing these nutrients. Increase the consumption of foods rich in iodine and reduce the intake of refined/processed foods. Be sure to use sea salt in cooking or sprinkled on foods as a source of iodine. A small dose (1/4 grain or less) of thyroid hormone may be necessary.

12 to 21 points *Moderately sluggish thyroid:* Severely curtail the consumption of refined sugar, since it causes thyroid burnout. Eat iodine-rich foods and be sure to salt your food with sea salt. Take the following supplements daily: tyrosine (1000 mg), B-complex (1 or 2 tablets), zinc (50 mg), and a multiple vitamin-mineral tablet containing iodine. A prescription of thyroid hormone (1/4 to 1/2 grain) may be necessary.

22 to 35 points *Severely sluggish thyroid:* At this level daily thyroid hormone replacement may be necessary. See your doctor and have him/her perform the appropriate blood tests for thyroid function. Be aware that the blood tests can be normal and a thyroid defect may still exist. That is because as much as 70% of thyroid function may be lost before blood tests become abnormal. If the physician suggests thyroid hormone therapy, opt for natural thyroid hormone versus synthetic (e.g. Synthroid), which may be toxic.

Certain substances impair thyroid function. These substances include refined sugar, fluoride, alcohol, hydrogenated fats, and caffeine. Additionally, a number of foods contain substances called goitrogens, which interfere with thyroid function. These anti-thyroid foods include raw cabbage, kale, cauliflower, broccoli, Brussels sprouts, beets, peanuts, almonds, peaches, flax, legumes, beans, carrots, and spinach. What's more, the anti-thyroid components are liberated by juicing. Ironically, the daily consumption of what is regarded to be a healthy food, raw carrot juice, may induce a mild hypothyroid state *(Note:* cooking inactivates the thyroid-blocking components). In order to reactivate thyroid function, take the following supplements on a daily basis:

- tyrosine - 2,000 mg daily
- iodine - 500 mcg daily
- riboflavin - 100 mg daily
- fat-soluble thiamine - 200 mg daily
- niacin - 200 mg daily
- vitamin B-6 - 50 mg daily
- zinc - 50 mg daily
- copper - 3 mg daily
- magnesium - 1,000 mg daily
- vitamin C - 2,000 mg daily

36 and above *Incompetent thyroid function:* Your thyroid gland is failing to work to any significant degree. To be certain that the symptoms are due to thyroid malfunction take the Broda Barnes underarm thyroid temperature test. This simple at-home test requires only a thermometer. Shake the thermometer down and place it at your bedside. As soon as you awaken put the thermometer under your armpit. Lay motionless in bed for ten minutes and then record the result. Do this for at least ten continuous days. The newer electronic thermometers require much less time. Women should be aware that their temperatures will naturally rise during

menses.   The normal underarm temperature is 97.8° or above.   If your temperature is consistently below this level, blood tests for evaluating thyroid function are indicated. However, be aware that these tests are often normal even if the thyroid gland is malfunctioning.   That is because the tests show only how much thyroid hormone is circulating in the blood and tell nothing of how well the hormones are functioning on a cellular level.   Additionally, the loss of up to 70% of thyroid function may occur before blood tests become abnormal.   The fact is thousands of Americans have thyroid glands which are operating at 10 to 30% capacity.   No wonder so many individuals suffer from chronic fatigue.

If the tests are abnormal, your doctor may suggest thyroid replacement therapy.   Insist upon natural thyroid hormone (Armor thyroid, etc.).   Do not take Synthroid. In addition, the following supplements should be consumed on a daily basis:

- tyrosine - 3,000 mg
- riboflavin - 100 mg
- fat-soluble thiamine - 300 mg
- magnesium - 1,000 mg
- iodine - 1 mg
- zinc - 50 mg
- copper - 3 mg
- niacin - 250 mg
- vitamin B-6 - 50 mg daily
- vitamin C - 3,000 mg daily
- selenium - 400 mcg daily

The Adrenal Failure Syndrome

The adrenal glands are the primary organ system for fighting stress. They are responsible for warding off the ill effects of every conceivable mental and/or physical stressor. Emotional strain causes a significant disruption of adrenal function. Anger is perhaps the most devastating of all mental stressors. Researchers have discovered that its negative effects on adrenal function are profound.

Virtually all patients with adrenal insufficiency suffer from severe allergic tendencies. The fact is these glands are the primary means for preventing or reversing allergic reactions. Adrenal failure is frequently associated with hypoglycemia. The adrenal glands exert potent control over blood sugar status and prevent the levels from dropping suddenly as a result of stress.   Individuals with weakened adrenal glands suffer from virtually all of the symptoms of the *Blood Sugar Collapse Syndrome* (see pp. 258-262).

The adrenal glands consist of two sections: an inner portion, known as the *medulla*, and an outer portion, known as the *cortex*.   The medulla produces adrenalin, while the cortex produces a complex array of steroid hormones, descriptively known as *cortical hormones*.   The latter category includes cortisone, DHEA (dihydroepiandosterone), aldosterone, progesterone, estrogen, and testosterone.

The adrenal glands, which are posed atop the kidneys, normally are golf-ball size. As a result of poor nutrition and/or stress, they may become significantly enlarged. This enlargement is due to a phenomenon known as *cellular hypertrophy*. Put simply, the cells within the adrenal glands multiply excessively in an attempt to supply the body with the additional steroid hormones demanded by stress. Poor nutrition compromises this process, since a wide range of nutriments are required for adrenal steroid synthesis to proceed normally.   The nutrients include fatty acids (especially cholesterol), amino acids, B-vitamins (especially pantothenic acid), vitamin E, vitamin A, vitamin C, bioflavonoids, zinc, selenium, potassium, sodium, manganese, chromium, and magnesium.   If the stresses remain unabated and the nutritional deficits are neglected, the adrenal glands ultimately self-destruct and shrink. This is known medically as *atrophy* of the adrenal cortex. When this adrenal atrophy becomes extreme, it may result in a potentially life-threatening condition called *Addison's disease*. In this instance the adrenal glands are totally incapable of producing steroid hormones. Individuals suffering with this condition are unable to cope with stress. Often the adrenal glands become so weak that even seemingly insignificant stresses can precipitate a decline in health.

Tens of millions of Americans suffer from the symptoms of adrenal insufficiency. This condition is rising in incidence every year largely due to the processed food diet. Severe emotional stress combined with extreme nutritional deficiencies are primary precipitating factors. Stress modification plus improved nutrition usually aids in regenerating the adrenal glands, resulting in return of normal function.

Which of these apply to you?

1. constant fatigue
2. muscular weakness
3. sweating or wetness of hands and feet
4. nervousness
5. fainting spells
6. chronic heartburn
7. alternating constipation and diarrhea
8. insomnia
9. low blood pressure
10. blood sugar disturbances
11. mood swings
12. paranoia
13. lightheaded sensation
14. headaches, particularly migraines
15. heart palpitations
16. cravings for salt
17. cravings for sweets
18. intolerance to alcohol

19. intolerance to cigarette smoke and/or exhaust fumes
20. hard pebble-like stools
21. vague indigestion
22. vague abdominal pain
23. vulnerability to food reactions/allergies
24. break out in hives or other rashes
25. clenching and/or grinding of teeth, especially at night
26. lack of appetite
27. infrequent urination and/or lack of thirst
28. premenstrual symptoms (PMS)
29. chronic pain in the lower neck and upper back
30. pain or tightness in the upper neck and/or scalp
31. inability to concentrate and/or confusion
32. panic attacks
33. phobias (agoraphobia, claustrophobia, etc.)
34. easily frustrated
35. compulsive behavior
36. intolerance to hot humid weather (heat exhaustion)
37. intolerance to cold and/or cold hands and/or feet
38. sense of well being after eating, especially supper
39. depression often relieved by eating
40. difficulty relaxing (unless working)
41. easily distracted
42. tendency to have guilt feelings
43. extreme sensitivity to odors and/or noises
44. inability to cope with stressful events
45. tendency to cry easily
46. clumsiness
47. Hair loss on the outer parts of the lower legs
48. Tightness of the armpits
49. Are you unusually ticklish?
50. Do you have upper back pain/tightness which worsens from stress or cold weather?
51. Do you have a lack of the sensation of fullness after eating?
52. Do you have fine thin hair?

53. Are your lower teeth (lower incisors) crowded, unequal in length, and/or misaligned?
54. Is your index finger longer than your ring finger?
55. Do you have a tendency to develop yeast or fungal infections?
56. Do you have a breathing disorder, particularly asthma?
57. Do you have an unusually small jaw bone or chin?
58. Have you taken cortisone pills (or prednisone) for prolonged periods (one month or longer)?
59. Do you drink caffeinated beverages on a daily basis?
60. Have you consumed large amounts of refined sugar throughout your life? (If so, add an additional 5 points to your score)
61. Do you consume alcoholic beverages on a daily basis?
62. Do you smoke 1 or more packs of cigarettes daily?
63. Do you have an excessively low cholesterol level (below 150 mg/dl)?
64. Do you regularly use cortisone creams or ointments?
65. Have you suffered or do you currently suffer from prolonged psychic/emotional stress?
66. Do you suffer from depression and/or weight gain during the winter months?
67. Were you regarded as a "lazy" child?
68. Are you or have you been frequently tormented or ridiculed by others?
69. Do you suffer from or have you suffered from severe infections, such as TB, blood poisoning, sepsis or hepatitis?
70. Do you have the initiative and desire to perform tasks but feel physically incapable of doing so?
71. Have you undergone numerous prolonged surgeries?
72. Are you jumpy and/or easily startled?
73. Do you have brown pigment spots about your temples, upper back, or chest?
74. Do you wet the bed or did you previously wet the bed?

75. Do you prefer hot drinks rather than cold drinks, or are you intolerant to cold drinks?

Your Score ____

1 to 11 points *Mild adrenal failure:* Even a mild state of adrenal failure can result in significant ill health. To correct this condition avoid substances toxic to the adrenal glands such as refined sugars, caffeine, cocoa, amphetamines, and alcohol. Follow a diet high in protein and natural fat and low in carbohydrates. Take 500 mg of pantothenic acid daily. Additionally, take a multiple vitamin plus minerals and extra vitamin C (1,000 to 2,000 mg daily). Salt your food to taste.

12 to 25 points *Moderate adrenal failure:* Warning—the adrenal failure will gradually worsen unless lifestyle and diet are altered. Worry, frustration, anxiety, and depression all create tremendous stress upon the endocrine system, with the adrenal glands bearing the brunt of the damage. Stop mentally battering your adrenal glands or risk falling into total adrenal failure.

The diet should be rich in protein and natural fats and low in sugars and starches. Complex carbohydrates, such as those found in brown rice, wild rice, potatoes, and coarse whole grains, may be well tolerated by some individuals. However, avoid all dietary sources of refined sugars and curb the consumption of foods naturally rich in sugar such as molasses, honey, fruit juices, oranges, pears, apples, etc.

Take the following supplements in order to preserve your adrenal function and repair any damage that has occurred:

pantothenic acid - 1,000 mg twice daily
B-complex - one tablet twice daily
vitamin C - 1,000 mg three times daily
licorice root extract - 2 or 3 capsules three times daily
tyrosine - 500 mg three times daily

vitamin A - 15,000 I.U. three times daily
potassium - 200 mg three times daily
chromium - 200 mcg three times daily
rice polishings - 3 heaping tablespoons daily

26 to 42 points   *Severe adrenal failure:* Beware—complete adrenal collapse is imminent. Lifestyle alterations must occur immediately, i.e. desist from worrying, fretting, grieving, and agitating. Depression and anxiety, as well as fits of anger, devastate adrenal function.

Curtail the consumption of all dietary sources of sugar and strictly adhere to a low-carbohydrate diet. Avoid all sources of alcohol and caffeine. In other words, eat primarily meats, nuts, seeds, olives, cheeses, vegetables, fish, and avocados. Be sure to snack on low-sugar/starch foods between meals to keep the blood sugar stable. Salty snacks such as roasted nuts, pickles, and cheese are ideal. For ideas on snacks and meals see my first book, *Eat Right to Live Long*. In addition, take the following nutritional aids:

pantothenic acid - 1,000 mg three times daily
B-complex - 1 tablet three times daily
vitamin C - 2,000 mg three times daily
tyrosine - 500 mg twice daily
vitamin E - 1200 I.U. daily
vitamin A - 25,000 I.U. twice daily
magnesium - 400 mg three times daily
selenium - 200 mcg three times daily
chromium - 250 mcg three times daily
manganese - 4 mg three times daily
licorice root - 3 capsules three times daily
potassium - 200 mg daily
coenzyme Q-10 - 100 mg daily
carnitine - 1 gram twice daily
rice polishings - 4 heaping tablespoons daily
Mexican yam extract - 3 capsules three times daily

Licorice root is an invaluable herb for the treatment of adrenal insufficiency. You may wish to drink a cup of licorice root tea each day. However, it is possible to consume it to an excess, and, like all herbs, licorice root possesses a certain degree of toxicity. As always, use moderation as the rule.

43 and above *Extreme adrenal failure:* You are in a state of complete adrenal collapse. Perhaps you knew you were ill but didn't realize why. Your adrenal glands are severely damaged, and, as a result, you are unable to cope with the basic elements of life itself. Immediately stop all behaviors and habits which disrupt adrenal function. If you smoke or drink, stop immediately. Curtail the consumption of all stimulants such as caffeine, cocoa, tea, and especially refined sugar. Refined sugar places great stress upon the adrenal glands, increasing the demand for the synthesis of various adrenal hormones. Sugar causes a wastage of adrenal hormones, and this may ultimately lead to internal bleeding within the glands and cellular death.

In order to reverse this pathological condition take the following supplements:

pantothenic acid - 2,000 mg three times daily
B-complex - 1 tablet three times daily
vitamin C - 2,000 mg three times daily
tyrosine - 500 mg three times daily
licorice root - 4 capsules three times daily
vitamin E - 1200 I.U. daily
vitamin A - 25,000 I.U. twice daily
magnesium - 400 mg three times daily
selenium - 200 mcg three times daily
chromium - 500 mcg three times daily
vitamin B-6 - 50 mg twice daily
potassium - 300 mg daily
bioflavonoids - 2 grams daily

coenzyme Q-10 - 100 mg twice daily
carnitine - 1 gram three times daily
rice polishings - 6 heaping tablespoons daily
gotu kola - 4 capsules daily
Mexican yam - 3 times daily

Remember, it took a number of years for you to arrive in your current state of health. Be patient; the adrenal glands will regenerate. However, it may take several months or even years before they heal completely.

Note: Individuals who score in the severe or extreme categories are candidates for hormone replacement therapy. Traditional sources of steroid hormones, such as hydrocortisone and prednisone, are toxic and should be avoided. Adrenal hormones which can be safely prescribed include DHEA (Dihydroepiandosterone), aldosterone, injectable adrenocortical extract, and natural source cortisol. Only nutritionally oriented doctors are likely to prescribe these. Progest cream is a non-prescription source of steroids. The active ingredient is an extract from a plant, the steroid-rich wild Mexican yam. Rub the cream twice daily on the large body parts, such as thighs, buttocks, breasts, or abdomen. For women vaginal administration offers optimal absorption. The cream also may be administered rectally.

The Blood Sugar Collapse Syndrome

Normally the blood contains sugar in the form of glucose. In fact, glucose is the primary cellular fuel. However, too little or too much sugar in the blood is dangerous. With an excess, diabetes develops. Usually, however, diabetes is preceded by a condition known as *hypoglycemia* or low blood sugar.

Blood sugar disorders are exceedingly common in the United States, with as many as one in two Americans being affected. This is primarily the result of the high sugar diet consumed by the majority of Americans.

The appropriate treatment of this condition is complicated by the fact that physicians are generally unaware that blood sugar disorders are a prevalent cause of ill health. Furthermore, the most accurate method for diagnosing blood sugar disorders, the six-hour glucose tolerance test, is only rarely performed by physicians even if a blood sugar disorder is suspected. To complicate matters the symptoms of blood sugar disorders occur in a wide variety of other illnesses. For example, depression, fatigue, and/or anxiety are among its most common symptoms. For these reasons the Blood Sugar Collapse Syndrome is the most underdiagnosed, as well as misdiagnosed, of all medical conditions in America today.

The brain consumes a greater amount of sugar for its weight than any other organ. The fact is the brain relies almost exclusively upon sugar, in the form of glucose, as its energy source. As a result, a sudden drop in the blood sugar level may lead to a variety of mental symptoms. Yet, disorientation, anxiety, anger, agitation, depression, and frustration are not the only problems that may arise from hypoglycemia. In fact, rather than developing mental symptoms, some individuals simply fall asleep and/or faint when their blood sugar collapses.

Which of these apply to you?

1. mood swings
2. fatigue after eating, worse if dessert is included
3. insomnia (especially waking up after falling asleep)
4. episodes of agitation or temper tantrums
5. dizziness and/or fainting spells
6. legs feel rubbery or weak
7. episodes of shakiness and/or tremors
8. clumsiness
9. headaches (worse after skipping a meal)

10. easily become upset and/or frustrated
11. episodes of cold sweats and/or nausea
12. disorientation
13. depression often relieved by eating
14. sleepiness after eating sugar, fruit, or starch
15. bursts of violent behavior and/or fits of anger
16. attention deficit (or childhood behavioral problems)
17. memory impairment or forgetfulness
18. paranoia and/or anxiety
19. crying spells
20. panic attacks
21. episodes of blurry vision
22. cantankerous behavior
23. sudden drop in energy level during mid-morning or mid-day
24. nightmares
25. constant worrying
26. indigestion
27. indecisiveness
28. sensations of impending doom
29. poor concentration
30. heart rhythm disturbances
31. uncontrollable negative or self-destructive thoughts
32. episodes of uncontrollable eating (binging)
33. episodes of sudden mental blackouts
34. Are you accident prone?
35. Do you constantly crave sweets and/or starches?
36. Do you drink alcohol heavily (two or more drinks per day)?
37. Do you consume sweets on a daily basis?
38. Do you have a history of liver and/or pancreatic disease?
39. Do you have a significant family history of diabetes?
40. Do you have chronic migraine headaches?
41. Do you eat fast food on a weekly basis (pizza, hot dogs, hamburgers, subs, doughnuts, etc.)?
42. Do you have intense cravings for salty foods?

43. Do you take birth control pills on a regular basis, or have you done so in the past for two years or more?
44. Have you taken large doses of cortisone, orally or injectable, or do you take it currently on a regular basis?

Your Score ____

1 to 9 points *Mild blood sugar collapse:* If untreated, your blood sugar problems will likely worsen with time. Remove all sources of refined sugars from the diet. Follow a diet rich in protein, natural fats, vegetables, and, to a lesser degree, complex carbohydrates. In addition, take a B-complex tablet and 100 mcg of chromium picolinate twice daily.

10 to 23 points *Moderate blood sugar collapse:* Treatment of this mentally and physically debilitating condition requires strict adherence to a low-sugar/starch diet (see *Eat Right To Live Long*). In addition, take the following supplements:

> chromium picolinate - 200 mcg three times daily
> biotin - 1 mg twice daily
> B-complex - 1 tablet twice daily
> zinc - 15 mg three times daily
> magnesium - 400 mg twice daily
> fat-soluble thiamine - 50 mg three times daily
> carnitine - 500 mg twice daily
> rice polishings - 2 heaping tbsp twice daily

Be sure to snack between meals. Safe snacks for blood sugar patients include raw vegetables, nuts, seeds, sliced fresh meats, chicken pieces, plain yogurt, avocados, and cheese.

24 and above *Severe blood sugar collapse:* Warning— continually abusing the body by consuming high-sugar foods and other highly processed foodstuffs could result in the onset of diabetes. Curtail the consumption of refined sugar and

reduce or eliminate sources of natural sugars such as honey, molasses, orange juice, apple juice, and fruit. Follow the aforementioned dietary advice, being sure to snack on high-protein or high-fat foods between meals. In addition, take the following supplements:

chromium picolinate - 200 mcg three times daily
manganese chelate - 2 mg three times daily
B-complex - one tablet twice daily
desiccated liver (organic) - 4 tablets twice daily
multiple mineral - 1 tablet three times daily
fat-soluble thiamine - 50 mg three times daily
zinc - 20 mg three times daily
biotin - 3 mg three times daily
magnesium - 400 mg twice daily
carnitine - 1 gram twice daily

The Yeast/Fungus Syndrome

Yeast and/or fungal infections have become one of the prominent plagues of Western civilization. This is largely a consequence of the Western diet. Fungi utilize primarily sugars and starches as their food. Their favorite "dish" is sugar. Fungal growth is most greatly enhanced by refined and/or heated sugar, although these organisms also efficiently feed on natural sugars such as those found in fruits and fruit juices.

The rampant use of antibiotics is an additional crucial factor which is responsible for the heightened incidence of yeast infections. Antibiotics kill only bacteria and are particularly aggressive in destroying the body's protective bacteria. This leaves the body vulnerable for colonization by yeasts and fungi.

The mucous membranes of the mouth, sinuses, lungs, intestines, uterus, urethra, and vagina are lined by untold billions of protective bacteria. When these bacteria are destroyed, the tissues are aggressively invaded by various yeast and fungi. This tissue invasion causes severe inflammation. Furthermore, the yeast/fungi produce highly toxic chemicals which disrupt immune function. In fact the chemicals are so powerful that the immune response against the yeast/fungi is essentially neutralized. Though the mucous membranes are the primary site of damage, chronic fungal infections of the internal organs may occur. The liver, spleen, kidneys, ovaries, thyroid gland, and adrenal glands are all susceptible to infection.

The majority of physicians regard antibiotics as being nontoxic. This is why they prescribe them repeatedly without concern and usually without warning patients of side effects. Patients take numerous doses with seeming impunity. Yet with each dose, the risk for chronic fungal infections is greatly accelerated. Other drugs which increase the risks for fungal infections include cortisone (especially prednisone), Tagamet, Zantac, antacids, and asthma medications. Tens of millions of Americans consume these drugs every year. Add to this the consumption of antibiotics, and the number of Americans regularly utilizing drugs which enhance fungal growth exceeds 50 million. It should be no surprise that as many as one in four Americans suffer ill health as a consequence of chronic fungal infection.

Fungi also commonly infect the skin. Sites which retain moisture are particularly vulnerable, such as between the toes, the scalp, the groin, and the umbilicus.

Which of these apply to you?

1. craving for sweets
2. low body temperature
3. indigestion or abdominal discomfort after eating fruits or other sweet foods
4. itching of the vagina, penis, groin, and/or rectum

5. rectal or vaginal burning
6. burning during or after urination
7. vaginal discharge (white, off-white, or cottage-cheesy)
8. skin and/or scalp itches after eating sugar and/or fruit
9. bloating after meals
10. persistent indigestion and/or heartburn
11. itching of the ear canals or umbilicus (belly button)
12. chronic sinus problems
13. intolerance to alcohol
14. sensitivity to chemicals, chemical odors, and/or cigarette smoke
15. seborrhea or heavy dandruff on the scalp, face, or hands
16. ringworm
17. itchy skin and/or scalp
18. reduced white blood count
19. constipation
20. feeling of being in a mental fog
21. chronic diarrhea
22. attention deficit
23. chronic sore or scratchy throat
24. "ice cold" hands or feet
25. severe intolerance to cold weather
26. Do you feel worse on damp humid days?
27. Do you have athlete's foot, toenail, or fingernail fungus?
28. Do you have a history of fungal infection of the internal organs, e.g. lungs, brain, kidneys, bladder, etc.?
29. Do you have a history of eczema and/or psoriasis?
30. Do you have an allergy or sensitivity to airborne molds?
31. Do you have a history of oral, rectal, and/or vaginal thrush?
32. Do you have painful menstrual cramps?
33. Do you have an allergy or sensitivity to moldy and/or fermented foods (blue cheese, aged cheeses, vinegar, soy sauce, brewer's yeast, baker's yeast, etc.)?
34. Do you consume refined sugar on a daily basis?

35. Do you take antibiotics daily, weekly, or monthly?
36. Have you taken ten or more courses of antibiotics (oral or IV) during your lifetime?
37. Do you consume large amounts of "natural sugars" on a daily basis, for instance, orange juice, apple juice, apples, bananas, raisins, pears, dates, prunes, prune juice, canned pineapple, pineapple juice, grape juice, etc.?
38. Do you eat commercially raised meats on a daily basis?
39. Do you have a history of ulcerative colitis or Crohn's disease?
40. Do you have a history of endometriosis?
41. Do you have recurrent urinary tract infections, i.e. bladder infections, urethritis, or pyelonephritis?
42. Do you use steroids (cortisone) on a regular basis (either orally, vaginally, on the skin, or as an inhalant)?
43. Do you use Tagamet, Zantac, and/or antacids regularly?

Your Score _____

1 to 8 points *Mild yeast infestation:* Reduce the consumption of refined sugars and restrict the intake of foods naturally high in sugars such as grapes, cherries, orange juice, apple juice, etc. Take an acidophilus supplement and/or eat unsweetened yogurt on a regular basis. Take immune-stimulating nutrients, such as vitamins A, C, E, B-5 and B-6, on a daily basis.

9 to 17 points *Moderate yeast infestation:* Follow the afore-mentioned advice. Certain nutrients help stimulate the immune system to destroy the yeast/fungus. The following immune-enhancing supplements are indicated:

selenium - 500 mcg
vitamin E - 800 I.U.
beta carotene - 50,000 I.U.

vitamin A - 25,000 I.U.
biotin - 5 mg
chromium - 400 mcg
vitamin C - 3,000 mg
manganese - 4 mg
vitamin B-6 - 30 mg
primrose oil - 6 capsules daily

Additionally, take an acidophilus supplement several times each day (frequent dosages increase the odds for implantation). Raw garlic and onions kill fungal organisms and should be consumed as often as possible. Supplemental garlic is also advised. Aloe vera juice and grapefruit seed extract also possess significant anti-fungal activity.

18 to 25 points *Severe yeast infestation:* Follow the previously mentioned advice regarding diet and supplements. Chronic yeast infections are a significant cause of ill health. Raw garlic and onions should be regularly included in the diet. Eat one clove of raw garlic every day for at least two weeks. Take immune system boosting herbs such as Pau D'arco, goldenseal root, echinacea, mullein, aloe, grapefruit seed extract, and astragalus. In addition, be sure to consume yogurt on a daily basis.

26 and above *Extreme yeast infestation:* At this phase of infestation it is possible that internal infection, that is infection of the internal organs, may exist. Destroy the yeasts with immunotherapy by taking the following nutrients:

beta carotene - 75,000 I.U.
vitamin A - 50,000 I.U.
selenium - 800 mcg
zinc - 70 mg
vitamin C - 4,000 mg
vitamin E - 800 I.U.

chromium - 400 mcg
magnesium - 4 mg
biotin - 5 mg
riboflavin - 50 mg
vitamin B-6 - 50 mg
folic acid - 10 mg

In addition, there are a host of herbs and other natural substances which kill fungi. They include grapefruit seed extract, aloe, goldenseal root, tannic acids, mathake, and Pau D'arco, any or all of which would be helpful additions to the anti-yeast protocol. Tanalbit, made by *Scientific Consulting Service*, is perhaps the most effective herbal anti-fungal agent available today. The appropriate dosage is usually 3 or 4 capsules taken morning, noon, and night. It may be ordered by calling (800) 243-5242.

Intestinal Parasite Syndrome

This is an exceedingly common syndrome, afflicting untold millions of Americans and hundreds of millions of people worldwide. Parasites may be defined as microbes which infect or "live off of" human tissue. The primary categorizations are *protozoans* and *helminths*. The protozoans include amoebas, giardia, and trichomonas. The helminths include the various worms such as roundworms, pinworms, hookworms, and tapeworms.

The major distinction between parasites and bacteria/viruses is that the former are larger and in some instances may become so large that they are visible with the naked eye. In contrast, bacteria and viruses can be seen only with the aid of a microscope. What makes parasites particularly danger-ous is that they can infect people via three forms: the live organism itself, its eggs, or its cysts.

Parasitic illnesses are a major plague of modern society. Both acute and chronic diseases may result from parasitic infections. Acute diseases include flu syndromes, hepatitis, food poisoning, diarrheal illness, appendicitis, and gallbladder attacks. Chronic diseases include anemia, colitis, intestinal ulcers, liver disease (including cirrhosis), arthritis, immune defects, and lung disease.

The "Milwaukee Parasite" crisis of 1993 is just one example of the enormity of this problem. In April 1993, this city's water supply was contaminated with a parasite called *cryptosporidium*. Apparently, the organism and/or its cysts are resistant to chlorine. It is estimated that some 400,000 people, or one half of the city's population, were infected; several died.

Parasites are often difficult to kill. The key is to stimulate the immune response against them. Additionally, various herbs are anti-parasitic, including black walnut extract, ginger root, echinacea, grapefruit seed extract, raw pumpkin seeds, garlic, oil of oregano, and onion extract.

Do you experience:

1. rectal itching
2. rectal pressure
3. muscular wasting and/or weakness
4. chronic vague abdominal pain
5. ravenous appetite
6. bloating, especially after eating
7. weight loss or inability to gain weight
8. constant or frequent heartburn
9. diarrhea
10. mucous in stools
11. night sweats
12. insomnia
13. severe fatigue
14. nausea and/or vomiting

15. fever and/or chills
16. constant belching
17. stomach pain after eating
18. poorly formed stools
19. itchy skin, worse at night
20. dark circles under the eyes
21. Have you traveled frequently overseas and/or to Mexico?
22. Have you ever developed diarrheal disease or severe fever while traveling abroad?
23. Do you frequently eat raw or smoked fish (sushi)?
24. Do you eat prosciutto and/or home-made sausages?
25. Do you own house dogs that you often handle, pet, or kiss?
26. Did you live overseas before becoming a U.S. resident?
27. Have you ever lived in a tropical region?
28. Do you drink untreated and/or unfiltered water in the wilderness or when traveling overseas?
29. Do you fail to wash your hands carefully after using the restroom?
30. Do you tend to experience digestive distress after eating fatty foods?
31. Do you have a long-term history of chronic anemia (low blood count)?

Your Score _____

1 to 6 points *Mild parasitic infestation:* Certain symptoms of parasitic infection are nonspecific. Thus, at this level the symptoms could be due to a variety of other illnesses or infections. As a trial to determine if you have parasites, eat 2 or 3 cloves of raw garlic daily. If the symptoms improve within one week, parasitic infestation is virtually confirmed.

7 to 14 points *Moderate parasitic infestation:* Medical tests for determining the presence of parasites are indicated. Eat two cloves of raw garlic three times daily, ideally on an

empty stomach (*Note:* Some individuals cannot tolerate this and should consume it only with meals.) If the symptoms improve, continue consuming 2 cloves three times daily for two weeks. Ideally, take the garlic while on a gallbladder/liver flush. The liver is a primary site of infestation, and the flush helps drive parasites from the liver into the bowels so that the garlic can destroy them. The flushing agent is a mixture of 1/4 to 1/2 cup of extra virgin olive oil (or pure rice bran oil) combined with several tablespoonfuls of vinegar or lemon juice. Drink this mixture three times daily. The flush should be performed for three to five days. During this period follow an exclusively high fat diet; your menu will consist of fatty foods such as eggs, cheese, butter, beef, lamb, avocados, olives, nuts, and seeds. Salads are allowed as are the following liver-cleansing fruits and vegetables:

black radish root
daikon and red radish
apple or pear skins (pectin binds toxins generated from
 the flush)
turnips
onions, garlic, leeks, shallots
parsley and watercress
capers
Jerusalem artichoke
citrus rind

Capers aid in liver regeneration; be sure to top your salads with them. Onions, garlic, turnips, and radishes are anti-parasitic in addition to being stimulants of biliary flow. However, the secret to the success of this flush is the olive oil and high-fat diet, since fat purges the liver of the bile and the parasites that live within it. Additionally, raw pumpkin seeds are anti-parasitic. Consume at least three large handfuls daily during the liver flush. Ginger root also possesses significant anti-parasitic activity: take 3 capsules three times daily on an empty stomach. Fresh ginger may also be used.

15 and above *Severe parasitic infestation:* Follow the advice listed previously. In addition, increase the garlic consumption during the liver flush to 4 cloves three times daily. Eat raw onions as often as possible. Take the various anti-parasitic herbs recommended previously and consume at least four handfuls of raw pumpkin seeds each day. Raw pumpkin seeds contain a substance which kills intestinal worms. A thymus glandular supplement (6 to 9 capsules), zinc (75 mg), and selenium (400 mcg) are crucial nutrients which provoke the anti-parasitic immune response. Additionally, try liquid Kyolic garlic as an immune stimulant, 2 tablespoons twice daily. *Intestinalis*, a doctor-formulated herbal anti-parasitic agent, may also prove useful: take 4 tablets three times daily. Oil of oregano is a potent anti-parasitic agent. Recently an emulsified oil of oregano product was made available by Biotics Research Corporation; take 2-3 tablets three times a day on an empty stomach.

The Inappropriate Estrogen Syndrome

Estrogen is regarded as essential to womanhood itself. While it is possible for women to live without it, the quality of their lives is usually compromised. However, estrogen deficiency is only one aspect of this dilemma. That is because many women have enough estrogen but suffer from a metabolic defect wherein they fail to utilize it properly. Other women produce an excess of estrogen, that excess being toxic. Abnormally high estrogen levels are associated with breast, uterine, and ovarian cancer in addition to less serious conditions such as cystic ovaries and fibrocystic breast disease. Oddly, the symptoms of too little, too much, and poorly utilized estrogen are similar, as is represented by this test.

271

Which of these apply to you?

1. night sweats
2. hot flashes
3. breast engorgement, worse during or before periods
4. insomnia
5. mood swings, worse during or before periods
6. heavy menstrual bleeding
7. excessive or painful menstrual cramps
8. dryness of the vaginal membranes
9. poor vaginal lubrication
10. PMS
11. loss of libido
12. Do you have a family history or current history of breast cancer?
13. Do you have a history of endometriosis?
14. Do you have a family history or current history of uterine fibroids?
15. Do you have a family history or current history of ovarian cysts?
16. Do you have a family history or current history of ovarian cancer?
17. Do you have a family history or current history of fibrocystic breast disease?
18. Do you take birth control pills?
19. Have you taken birth control pills for 5 or more years in the past?
20. Have you undergone a complete or partial hysterectomy?
21. Do you become weak or tired prior to or during menses?
22. Do you suffer from headaches occurring prior to or during menses?
23. Do you suffer from hirsutism (i.e. excessive hair growth), especially on the face?
24. Do you maintain excessive amounts of weight in your hips and/or breasts?

25. Do you suffer from chronic liver disease?
26. Do you consume refined sugar on a daily or weekly basis?
27. Do you consume margarine, refined vegetable oils, and/or deep-fried foods on a daily basis?
28. Do you consume alcohol and/or caffeine on a daily basis?
29. Do you have a history of infertility and/or repeated miscarriages?
30. Do you adhere to a strict low-fat diet?
31. Have you had an abnormal pap smear, or do you suffer from cervical dysplasia?

Your Score _____

1 to 6 points *Mild estrogen imbalance:* This low-level imbalance is probably due to a metabolic defect rather than a deficiency/excess. The metabolism of estrogen is controlled by the liver, ovaries, and adrenal glands, and it is likely that the function of these organs is impaired. Additionally, B-vitamins help regulate estrogen synthesis and metabolism. Correct this imbalance by taking a B-complex supplement and by following a diet rich in natural fats as well as cholesterol. Estrogen is a cholesterol molecule and, thus, dietary choles-terol is an important resource for its synthesis. In addition, take 5 mg of folic acid each day, since this B-vitamin is the primary one for regulating estrogen synthesis. Avoid refined sugar, alcohol, caffeine, and strictly avoid the consumption of refined oils.

6 to 13 points *Moderate estrogen imbalance:* Follow the pre-viously mentioned advice. In addition, take large doses of the nutrients which stimulate and/or regulate estrogen production, as follows:

    folic acid - 5 to 10 mg
    riboflavin - 50 mg

vitamin B-6 - 50 mg
choline - 1 gram
magnesium - 800 mg
pantothenic acid - 1 gram
vitamin E - 1200 I.U.
vitamin A - 50,000 I.U.

14 and above *Severe estrogen imbalance:* At this level of imbalance estrogen replacement therapy may be indicated. However, most estrogenic drugs are toxic, and evidence exists that women who take them over prolonged periods have a higher risk for breast and/or uterine cancer. Estriol is a nontoxic form of estrogen but is not readily available from traditional pharmacies. The solution may be to take herbs which stimulate the production of estrogen as well as the vitamins that increase its synthesis. Herbs that aid in the production of estrogen include:

ginger	fennel seed
dong quai	unicorn root
licorice root	wheat germ extract
Mexican yam	(octascosanol)
sarsaparilla	gotukola

Note: The symptoms of Inappropriate Estrogen Syndrome may be due primarily to progesterone deficiency. A deficiency of this hormone occurs most commonly premenstrually. Progesterone can be taken with greater safety than estrogen. A natural type of progesterone is available under the brand name *Progest.* Its active ingredient is an extract of the Mexican yam, which is a rich source of sex hormones. *Progest* is available as a cream or sublingual drops.

The Liver Dysfunction Syndrome

The liver is the body's workhorse, performing a greater number of functions than any other organ. In particular the liver is responsible for the detoxification of any external poisons as well as those produced within the body. Diseases of the liver are occurring with an alarmingly high frequency. Such diseases include liver cancer, hepatitis, Gilbert's disease, liver abscesses, parasitic infestation, diabetes, and cirrhosis.

Alcoholism is rampant, and as many as 30 million Americans suffer liver damage as a result of constant abuse. Alcoholics constitute a greater number of addicted individuals than all heroin, marijuana, cocaine, and prescription drug addicts combined. Alcoholics pay a heavy price for chronic consumption. As many as a million liver cells, as well as brain cells, are destroyed by a single alcoholic drink. It should be no surprise that alcohol is the number one cause of liver disease. Yet, heavy damage is inflicted upon other organs as well. Alcohol is a primary cause of hypertension, stroke, pancreatic disease, and heart disease as well as numerous types of cancer.

Long-term consumption of alcohol causes extensive liver damage, ultimately resulting in hepatitis and cirrhosis. Hepatitis is a potentially life-threatening disease. Alcohol consumption is one of many causes of hepatitis. Infectious hepatitis may develop as a result of inappropriate hygiene and sanitation, the consumption of foul water, or food contamination (for instance, shellfish contaminated by water-borne feces). Chemical hepatitis may occur as the result of drug/ alcohol addiction, toxic chemical exposure poisoning, and drug reactions. Additionally, hepatitis can be transmitted during sex and, in fact, occurs most commonly in the sexually promiscuous.

The liver marshals several essential functions. It acts as the primary storage depot for nutrients: vitamins, minerals, antioxidants, and co-enzymes. The synthesis of various proteins occurs primarily in the liver, including the crucial antioxidant enzymes, such as glutathione and superoxide dismutase. Additionally, it aids in the metabolism of a variety of hormones, including thyroid hormone, estrogen, and adrenal steroids. Finally, the liver is the primary organ responsible for the detoxification and decomposition of molecular compounds, whether natural or synthetic. For instance, it is the only organ which can efficiently rid the body of the breakdown products of commonly consumed substances, such as alcohol, drugs, fat-soluble vitamins, preservatives, artificial colors/ flavors and/or hormones.

All obese individuals suffer from impaired liver function. That is because the liver is the first internal organ to become infiltrated with fat. The fat is deposited within the liver cells, which are known as *hepatocytes*, greatly impairing their ability to function. In the extreme this fat infiltration causes balloon degeneration of the liver cells or, put simply, cellular death. Usually, when the weight is lost the liver cells regenerate and function returns to normal. In addition, certain nutrients, notably biotin, lipoic acid, thiamine, inositol, choline, and methionine, aid in liver cell regeneration by reversing fatty liver.

This exam is applicable to those suffering from extensive liver disease as well as individuals whose livers simply aren't working up to speed. The liver is the human body's primary detoxification organ, and it processes billions of molecules of noxious agents every hour of every day. Therefore, it is crucial to keep the liver in an optimal a state of health.

Which of these apply to you?

1. intolerance to alcohol
2. intolerance to sugar
3. tendency to gain weight easily
4. blood sugar disturbances

5. pale, greasy stools that float
6. chronic indigestion unrelieved by antacids
7. intolerance to fatty foods and/or cooking oils
8. foul-smelling bowel gas
9. sensitivity to chemical fumes (exhaust fumes, diesel fumes, perfumes, etc.)
10. high cholesterol and/or triglycerides (or excessively low cholesterol - below 140 mg/dl)
11. persistent sleepiness (narcolepsy) and/or fatigue
12. sudden hair loss
13. right-sided upper abdominal pain
14. chronic itching (pruritus)
15. dark circles and/or bags under the eyes
16. Do you consume alcohol regularly (4 or more drinks per week)?
17. Are you 20 or more pounds overweight?
18. Do you have a history of hepatitis and/or cirrhosis?
19. Do you have a history of intestinal or hepatic parasites?
20. Do you consume Tylenol on a daily or weekly basis?
21. Has your gallbladder been removed, and/or do you have a history of gallstones?
22. Do you have chronic constipation (fewer than one bowel movement per day)?
23. Do you take two or more prescription medications on a daily basis?
24. Have you in the past or do you currently use recreational or hard drugs (marijuana, cocaine, heroine, etc.)?
25. Have you received or are you currently receiving chemotherapy treatments?
26. Are you taking cholesterol-lowering medications?
27. Do you work with or near toxic chemicals, or have you worked with them in the past?
28. Do you have elevated bilirubin and/or liver enzymes?
29. Do you have a history of impaired immunity and/or immune deficiency?
30. Do you have thick ridges on the fingernails?

31. Do you take birth control pills, or have you taken them for one year or longer in the past?
32. Do you have a low blood globulin level?
33. Are you a diabetic, or do you have a significant family history of diabetes?
34. Do you have a tendency to bleed excessively (poor blood clotting)?
35. Do you have giardia infection, intestinal worms, or amoebic dysentery?

Your Score _____

1 to 7 points *Mild liver dysfunction:* Mild dysfunction of the liver can usually be resolved through dietary means and by avoiding toxic compounds. Increase the consumption of liver-detoxifying foods such as onions, garlic, leeks, shallots, capers, radishes, turnips, dark greens, squash, and pumpkin. Avoid refined vegetable oils, drugs, alcohol, and refined sugars.

8 to 14 points *Moderate liver dysfunction:* The liver is the human body's manufacturing plant. It is crucial to optimize liver function to prevent disease and improve health. Avoid direct contact with toxic compounds in or around the home or at work. Sugar tends to impair liver function. Thus, high carbohydrate foods, such as pasta, breads, sweets, and bakery, should be avoided. Hydrogenated oils impair liver function. Avoid them entirely. Consume foods which aid in liver detoxification such as ginger root, parsley, parsley root, radishes, watercress, cilantro, and onions. In addition to dietary changes, take the following supplements:

beet juice tablets or powder
dandelion root - 6 capsules daily
organic selenium - 300 mcg daily
beta carotene - 25,000 I.U. daily

fat-soluble thiamine - 200 mg daily
choline and methionine - 1 gram of each daily
acidophilus and bifidus - 2 capsules of each twice daily
biotin - 3 mg twice daily

15 to 21 points   *Severe liver dysfunction:* It is crucial to change dietary habits immediately.   Refined vegetable oils, margarine, partially hydrogenated fats, and refined sugars are all hepatotoxic.   Curtail the consumption of alcoholic beverages, and, if you are taking drugs, do everything possible to reduce the dosage.   Preferably, work with your doctor to eliminate them.   Additionally, follow the gallbladder/liver flush suggested in the section on parasitic infestation. Take the following supplements on a daily basis:

beet juice powder or tablets
dandelion root - 8 capsules
selenium - 500 mcg
beta carotene - 50,000 I.U.
vitamin E - 800 I.U.
silymarin - 1 gram
choline and methionine - 1 gram of each
biotin - 5 mg twice daily
inositol - 1 gram twice daily
vitamin C - 2,000 mg
ginger - 6 capsules
Kyolic garlic (with lecithin) - 4 capsules twice daily
acidophilus and bifidus - 3 capsules with meals
chlorella or spirulina - several capsules daily

23 and above *Extreme liver dysfunction:* Warning—continued exposure to toxic chemicals, drugs, or alcoholic beverages may cause irreparable liver damage.   Blood tests for determining liver function are definitely indicated.

Follow the previously mentioned dietary advice.   Drink no alcohol.   Consume foods which stimulate the healing processes within the liver. Examples include black and daikon radishes, onions, garlic, leeks, turnips, beets, watercress, parsley, raw nuts/seeds, ginger, turmeric, and capers. Try the Gingerized Liver Regeneration Drink in the recipe section (see Appendix B). In addition, take the following liver-repairing supplements on a daily basis:

beet juice tablets or powder
selenium - 600 mcg
choline and methionine - 1 gram of each
biotin - 10 mg twice daily
inositol - 2 grams twice daily
vitamin E - 1200 I.U.
dandelion root -10 capsules
silymarin - 1 gram
black radish root - 8 capsules
beta carotene - 50,000 I.U.
ginger - 9 capsules daily
fat-soluble thiamine - 500 mg
vitamin C - 2,000 mg
Kyolic garlic (with lecithin) - 4 capsules twice daily
acidophilus and bifidus - 3 capsules twice daily
chlorella or spirulina - several capsules daily
Livit-2 - 3 tablets three times daily

A number of products are available specifically formulated for the regeneration of damaged liver tissue. Many of these products consist of a specific combination of herbs. Livit-2 is an herbal formula which has been shown in clinical studies to help reduce the levels of elevated liver enzymes and return liver function to normal. Modified fasting programs have also been determined to be of value in inducing a remission in toxic liver syndromes.

The Malabsorption Syndrome

Malabsorption is defined as the inability to absorb nutrients from the food into the blood. Millions of Americans suffer from this condition, many unknowingly.

The digestive tract consists of numerous organs, all of which perform their own unique functions for the breakdown of food and absorption of nutrients. These organs include the stomach, small intestine, large intestine, pancreas, and liver. Defective function of any one of these organs can result in malabsorption.

Nutrients are absorbed primarily in the small intestine. This organ contains a delicate lining consisting of billions of microscopic organ systems called *intestinal villi*. These villi control the absorption of nutrients from the intestine into the bloodstream. Deficiency of certain nutrients, notably zinc and folic acid, leads to the destruction of intestinal villi.

Food allergy is perhaps the most common cause of malabsorption. A dramatic example is allergy to grains (gluten intolerance), which may lead to wholesale destruction of the intestinal villi. Other primary causes include intestinal parasitic infection, enzyme deficiency, intestinal bacterial flora imbalance, alcoholism, and reduced stomach acid output (hypochlorhydria).

In severe cases malabsorption leads to widespread nutritional deficiencies. The problem may become so extreme that certain individuals develop deficits of virtually every major nutrient. Not surprisingly, a variety of deficiency-induced illnesses, such as osteoporosis, lung disease, Chronic Fatigue Syndrome, immune deficiency, emaciation, Crohn's disease, arthritis, anemia, and liver disease, are associated with chronic malabsorption.

Which of these apply to you?

1. excessive weight loss or gain
2. greasy foul-smelling stools
3. hair loss and/or balding
4. constipation, particularly from eating certain foods
5. chronic diarrhea
6. undigested food in the stool
7. bloating and indigestion after meals unrelieved by antacids
8. foul-smelling intestinal gas
9. belching after meals
10. chronic heartburn
11. premature graying of the hair
12. hangnails
13. ridges on the nails and/or brittle nails
14. dry flaky and/or chapped skin
15. chronic fatigue
16. blood sugar disturbances
17. tendency to develop cavities
18. seborrhea and/or severe dandruff
19. geographic tongue and/or bald spots on the tongue
20. red or inflamed tongue
21. Has your stomach been surgically removed?
22. Has a portion of your intestines been surgically removed?
23. Do you take antacids on a daily basis?
24. Do you take Zantac or Tagamet on a daily basis?
25. Do you consume alcohol on a daily basis?
26. Are you a diabetic, or do you suffer from hypoglycemia?
27. Do you have lactose or milk intolerance?
28. Do you have an active intestinal or stomach ulcer?
29. Do you take laxatives, including mineral and castor oil, on a daily or weekly basis?
30. Do you have a history of celiac disease or gluten intolerance?

31. Do you have liver or pancreatic disease?
32. Do you have cystic fibrosis?
33. Do you have a history of Crohn's disease, ulcerative colitis, or irritable bowel syndrome?
34. Are you undergoing chemotherapy treatments?
35. Do you suffer from systemic skin diseases such as psoriasis, eczema, and dermatitis?
36. Do you have a history of intestinal parasitic infection?
37. Are you anemic?
38. Do you take antibiotics on a daily or weekly basis?

Your Score _____

1 to 7 points   *Mild malabsorption:* The symptoms of malabsorption are often vague. However, for preventive insurance you should consider undergoing food allergy testing, since the primary cause of malabsorption is food intolerance. In my experience the finest food allergy test available for discovering foods which cause malabsorption is performed by Nutritional Testing Labs. The address for the lab is Tower II, 1701 Golf Road (Suite 606), Rolling Meadows, Illinois, 60008. The cost is $450.00 for 204 foods or approximately $2.00 per food. The laboratory's phone number is (708) 640-1377. This test offers a significantly greater degree of accuracy than other allergy tests such as scratch, RAST, and ELISA tests. It is also of value for individuals suffering from asthma, arthritis, lupus, irritable bowel syndrome, and migraine headaches, all of which are due primarily to food allergy reactions.

8 to 16 points   *Moderate malabsorption:* Be sure to chew foods thoroughly. Consider having a Food Intolerance Test performed. Certain condiments stimulate the flow of digestive juices, including hot/tangy spices and vinegar. Use vinegar on all salads and add prodigious quantities of spices to your foods. Take 5 mg of folic acid twice daily. Increase the intake

of predigested foods such as yogurt, kefir, tempeh, and raw honey.

17 and above *Severe malabsorption:* Warning—significant nutritional deficiencies are occurring as a result of intestinal malabsorption. It is virtually assured that food allergies are the major culprit, and, thus, food intolerance testing is indicated. Pancreatic insufficiency and gluten intolerance are also likely. If you also scored high on the test for intestinal parasites, this may be the primary cause of the malabsorption. In addition to following the previously mentioned advice, take the following supplements:

    lactobacillus - as indicated by the package directions
      (or take 2 capsules before every meal)
    digestive enzymes - 3 with each meal and an additional
      3 one hour after meals
    folic acid - 5 mg twice daily
    zinc - 50 mg daily
    vitamin B-6 - 50 mg daily
    B-complex - 1 tablet daily
    multiple mineral - 2 tablets daily
    ginger root - 3 capsules with every meal
    aloe vera juice - 2 ounces twice daily
    chlorella - add packet of granules to each dose of aloe
      vera juice

Remember, the cure is efficiently achieved only if the cause is determined, whether food allergies, parasitic infection, yeast infection, or pancreatic disease. If the condition fails to improve, see your physician.

Achieving Optimal Results

By reading this book the majority of individuals have received a startling revelation: they are deficient in a variety of nutrients. True, the nutritional recommendations in this book are extensive and may appear complex to some. Do not feel overwhelmed by the recommendations of various vitamin/mineral supplements. The first step is to change your diet and lifestyle. Next, purchase a quality multiple vitamin-mineral product. Men and post-menopausal women must buy iron-free multiple vitamins. If B-vitamin deficiencies are major weak areas, purchase a B-complex supplement. Start with these as a foundation, then add additional nutrients based on the severity of the deficiencies. For instance, if you are deficient in all of the B-vitamins but severely deficient in two of them, for instance, folic acid and B-6, then you should take additional doses of these two B-vitamins combined with whatever is found in your B-complex pill. Use the same method for supplementing minerals.

Always remember that the finest sources for vitamins and minerals are organically grown foods. Thus, the resolution of nutritional deficiency ideally would be accomplished through dietary correction, that is through the consumption of organically produced fruits, vegetables, milk products, grains, and meats. Soup made with organically raised foods is an excellent way to achieve this; the broth is extremely rich in vitamins and minerals. Additionally, supplement the diet with nutrient-dense foods (see page 300). However, diet alone rarely suffices for resolving severe nutritional deficits. Supplements play a major role here.

The ancillary nutrients, such as antioxidants, enzymes, fatty acids, and coenzymes, may need to be supplemented individually. Everyone living in an industrialized or urban region would benefit from consuming extra vitamin E, beta carotene (vitamin A), and vitamin C besides what is received in the diet. Essential fatty acid deficiency is so common in the United States that routine consumption of a natural fatty acid supplement would be the rule rather than the exception. Digestive enzyme deficiency is also exceedingly common. A variety of enzyme supplements are available in the marketplace made from both animal and plant sources. If the various aforementioned specialty nutritional products are unavailable in your area, you may order them by calling Nutritional Supplement Service, 800-243-5242.

Food sources of the nutrients mentioned in this book are listed in Appendix A, but only the top sources are included. These foods will be of the greatest value for aggressive correction of long-standing nutritional deficiencies.

Conclusion

Tens of millions of people throughout the globe suffer ill health as a consequence of nutritional deficiencies. Individuals reading this book may be surprised to find themselves among the victims. A greater number of people will fail the exams than those who will pass them.

Currently, nutritional deficiency is equally common in the Western World and the Third World. This was thoroughly proven early in this century, notably by the work of Weston Price, DDS. Price traveled throughout the world, visiting both civilized and primitive societies. His work is immortal, since many of the primitive societies he studied are no longer in existence. Price clearly documented the fact that Americans suffer from a wide range of nutritional deficiencies as well as diseases unheard of in most primitive civilizations. His book, *Physical Degeneration*, makes fascinating reading, complete with photographs, and is available from the Price-Pottenger Foundation (see Appendix C).

An individual does not have to develop beriberi or scurvy to have a nutritional deficiency. Virtually all Americans suffer from the consequences of nutrient deficits. Recent surveys show that the average American gets significantly less than the RDA for a variety of nutrients, including vitamins A, C, and E, magnesium, folic acid, riboflavin, pyridoxine, pantothenic acid, chromium, manganese, copper, selenium, and zinc. Plus, Americans consume excessive amounts of low-nutrient foods such as white flour, white rice, white sugar, and margarine. As many as 70% of dietary calories may be derived from such devitalized foodstuffs.

Certain individuals, including many nutritional "authorities," maintain that Americans get all the nutrients they need from their food. These individuals claim that the body's nutritional needs are entirely met as a result of the fact that Americans regularly consume foods from all four food groups such as commercial fruits and vegetables. As such, the "experts" are unwilling to accept the undeniable facts: frozen and canned vegetables and fruits exhibit nutrient losses ranging from 20 to 95%. For instance, these experts are apparently unaware that supermarket citrus fruit is usually gas ripened and that often the fruit contains no measurable amounts of vitamin C. Michael Colgan, Ph.D., proved this at the Rockefeller institute over a decade ago. Yet, it is not common knowledge that fresh fruit is no longer a top vitamin C source.

To make matters worse, orthodox nutritionists and Americans in general are unaware of the differences between organic food and commercially grown food. How many people realize that an organically grown tomato may contain a tenfold or even greater magnesium content than a commercially grown one and that it may contain three times the vitamin C and twice the vitamin A? What's more, organic tomatoes taste better. The point is that the current generation is getting significantly less vitamins and minerals in their food, even in fresh produce, than did people living in the era preceding modern chemical farming. A reasonable estimate is that people today receive less than one-third of the minerals our ancestors did prior to 1950. As a result, mineral deficiency is rampant in the USA.

The dilemma of widespread nutritional deficiency is not solved by food fortification. In fact, this process solves few problems and may actually create additional ones. Relatively few vitamins are added to foods, and the only foods which are fortified are products containing white flour, refined corn, or white rice (milk products are also vitamin-fortified). What's more, the vitamin/mineral mix added by food processors contains a toxin: inorganic iron. This form of iron binds to and inactivates certain nutrients, notably vitamin E and vitamin C. Thus, inorganic iron is a nutrient robber, not a fortifier. White rice and flour are lacking in dozens of nutrients. What good is accomplished by the addition of a few milligrams of B-vitamins and inorganic iron when dozens of other nutrients are missing? The original food quality cannot be resurrected by such an incomplete approach. In fact, a good rule to follow is that if a food has been fortified, avoid it. Milk products may be an exception, since they are fortified with vitamin D and most of us could use extra amounts of this nutrient.

The nutritional tests in this book allow people to gain a better idea of the degree to which they are nutritionally deficient. However, this knowledge is valueless unless it is acted upon. If no action is taken, the deficiencies will only deepen with time, and the risks for degenerative diseases will rise correspondingly. On the other hand, if the diet is altered and measures for corrective supplementation are applied, improved health will result.

If you are healthy, use the self-tests in this book as a means to fine tune your health so that you may remain healthy for your entire lifetime. Ninety days after beginning a corrective program, repeat those tests on which you scored poorly. This will help in monitoring your improvement. A significant reduction in symptoms, for instance, dropping from a severe to a mild category, is a signal that you are "on the right track." Above all, do not procrastinate. No one can afford the prospect of ill health, since it may be difficult for the individual to rebuild his/her health once it has deteriorated.

The health status of the body and mind are linked inseparably. The fact is, our minds are affected by what we eat or fail to eat. The function of the body and mind will improve as a consequence of nutritional revitalization. Who wouldn't wish to have a greater degree of strength and energy, enhanced beauty, serenity and happiness, and a sharper-thinking mind? These benefits will automatically occur with improved nutrition.

The brain requires nutrients, and if it gets less than its share, all sorts of symptoms are possible: headaches, mental fatigue, memory loss, depression, apathy, anxiety, agitation, anger, mood swings, suicidal thoughts, and even violent behavior. The body revolts when it is fed poorly and when it is deprived of essential nutrients. The results are: fatigue, pain, digestive distress, and, ultimately, disease.

No one wants to live his/her later years like an invalid, as so many do today. Nursing homes and mental hospitals are filled to capacity. The occupants uniformly live a poor quality of life. Sadly, their health is so defective that they can no longer care for themselves. Such individuals are grossly deficient in a wide range of nutrients, and there is little they can do about it. In fact, the bland diet nursing home residents receive only deepens the extent of their nutritional deficiencies. Unfortunately, instead of correcting the deficiencies, physicians prescribe drugs which accelerate nutrient loss and impair the absorption of vitamins and minerals.

Nursing home patients struggle to survive each day. Most people would rather be dead than to live this way. Hospitalized patients are in no better condition, nutritionally speaking. The same pasty, empty-nutrient diet is fed to them as well.

As a rule, institutionalized food is tasteless, starchy, nutritionally depleted, and overcooked. It is as if bland food is the determinant for how good it is for you. What is the nutritional value of twice overcooked oatmeal, white bread, saltines, pastries, puddings, biscuits, instant potatoes, white rice, gravies, canned fruit, Jello, canned vegetables, extra well done meats, margarine, muffins, jelly, cane sugar, and 7-Up? It is nil.

As an example of the extensive nutritional ignorance of the medical profession, one of the most noxious of all foodstuffs, deep fried foods, is still on the menu in all hospitals. Whole grains are an anomaly. As for fresh fruits and vegetables, they are a rare delicacy. Hospital dietitians plan menus as though they have no clue as to what a nutritionally competent diet is, and they are entirely unaware of the fact that nutritional deficiencies in hospitalized patients are rampant. The food not only tastes bad but is bad for you, especially if you are already sick.

If you are fortunate enough to possess good health, the knowledge you have gained from reading this book can be applied for prevention, that is for keeping your body and mind fit and strong. If you are ill, you have an ideal opportunity to correct the nutritional deficits and dietary excesses which may be contributing to your condition.

Fatigue is not an inevitable consequence of aging nor is memory loss, hunched posture, chronic pain, hearing loss, and wrinkled skin. If nutritional deficiencies can be discovered early enough and corrected aggressively, the aging process can be stalled or even reversed. Thus, it is possible to feel good and look vital despite the acceleration of years.

The diet is simple. Avoid all toxins and processed foods listed in the self-tests. Eat wholesome foods and avoid any foods to which you are allergic. Steer clear of food faddism. Instead, concentrate on the invigorating value of all of the God-given foods: fruits, vegetables, fresh meats, eggs, dairy products, nuts, seeds, and whole grains.

Persistence is the key to nutritional correction. Following the diet temporarily or taking the nutrients for only a few days won't resolve the problem. It took a long time for the individual to get in his/her current condition, and it will take many days, weeks, or months for the full benefits of rehabilitation to be realized. Take your nutritional supplements regularly, preferably two or three times daily, and religiously follow a nutritious diet. As a result of this persistence you can achieve the immense benefits of improved nutrition: better health, improved vitality, enhanced mental acuity, increased strength, and a fuller, longer life.

Appendix A

Dietary Sources of Nutrients

Top Sources of Vitamin A

cod liver oil
liver (calf, lamb, beef)
pumpkin
parsley
hot red chili peppers
carrot juice
apricots, dried or raw
sweet potatoes
chlorella and spirulina
collards
beet greens
kale
winter squash
watercress
broccoli
escarole
pimentos
persimmons
halibut
salmon
peaches, dried or raw
butter

paprika
alfalfa leaf meal
carrots
parsley juice
dandelion greens
sea plasma
turnip greens
spinach
Swiss chard
butternut squash
asparagus
endive
arugula
capers
crab
oysters
swordfish
cantaloupe
egg yolks
tomato juice
nectarines

Top Sources of Vitamin B-12

liver (beef or lamb)
kidneys
haddock
cod
clams
eggs
mozzarella cheese
catfish
salmon
red meats

herring
fish eggs (from herring,
  cod, or mackerel)
crab
oysters (raw)
sardines
tuna
chlorella
spirulina

Top Sources of Vitamin B-6

rice bran
sunflower seeds
torula yeast
brewer's yeast
wheat germ and bran
parsley, dried
tuna
beef or lamb liver
walnuts
soybean flour
salmon mackerel
chicken (white meat is best)

brown rice
bananas
whey
fresh sweet corn
halibut
Brazil nuts
peanuts
fresh peanut butter
almonds
pecans
hazelnuts

Top Sources of Vitamin C

acerola berries
rose hips
Spanish orange
coriander leaf, dried
hot chili peppers
chili powder
guavas
strawberries
oranges
grapefruits
lemons
turnip and beet greens
mustard greens
parsley (raw)
broccoli

lamb's quarters
kale
collards
cabbage (red)
papaya
spinach
kiwi fruit
red sweet peppers
lemon or lime juice
orange juice
grapefruit juice
tomato juice
watercress
Swiss chard

Top Sources of Vitamin D

herring
sardines
mackerel
salmon
tuna
fish eggs (roe)
cod liver or cod liver oil

egg yolks
beef or lamb liver
cream
butter
cheese
whole milk
  (vitamin D-fortified)

Top Sources of Vitamin E

wheat germ oil
sunflower oil
avocado oil
soy bean oil
almond oil
extra virgin olive oil
wheat germ (raw)
hazelnuts
hazelnut oil
safflower oil
shrimp and lobster
brown rice
avocados

Brazil nuts
peanuts
fresh peanut butter
pecans
asparagus
red meat
organ meats
sweet potatoes
egg yolks
salmon and tuna
almonds
cabbage
spinach

Top Sources of Vitamin K

green tea
beet greens
kohlrabi
kale
cauliflower
alfalfa meal
cabbage
fresh red meats
spinach
watercress

cheese
oats
turnip greens
broccoli
lettuce
beef or lamb liver
asparagus
coffee
butter
Brussels sprouts

Top Sources of PABA

eggs
liver
wheat germ
soybeans

lecithin
peanuts
blackstrap molasses

Top Sources of Thiamine

brewer's yeast
torula yeast
red muscle meats
organ meats
rice bran
wheat germ
sunflower seed flour

sunflower seeds
pine nuts (or piñon)
soybean flour
sesame seeds
coriander leaf, dried
Brazil nuts
oat bran

Top Sources of Riboflavin

liver (beef and lamb)
kidney
brewer's yeast
cheese
whey
whole milk (fresh)

mushrooms (raw)
almonds
turnip greens
wheat bran
soybean flour
eggs

Top Sources of Niacin

brewer's yeast
liver and kidney
beef
chicken
lamb
turkey
rabbit
mushrooms
tuna
rice bran
instant coffee
rice polishings

wheat bran and germ
peanuts or peanut butter
paprika
salmon
mackerel
halibut
trout
pheasant
quail
tomato paste
green peas
brown rice

Top Sources of Pantothenic Acid

brewer's yeast
torula yeast
whey
rice polishings
brown rice
rice bran
egg yolks
kidney
butter milk
wheat bran
beef heart

peanut butter
peanuts
mushrooms
soybean flour
salmon
blue cheese
pecans
beans
buckwheat flour
sesame seeds
tahini

Top Sources of Folic Acid

organ meats
rice bran
rice germ
egg yolks
soybean flour
chicken (dark meat)
spinach (raw)
liver
endive (curly or escarole)
parsley (raw)
almonds
peanuts
fresh peanut butter
cabbage (raw)
beets and beet tops
cauliflower

broccoli
Brie cheese
cottage cheese
spinach
sour cream
powdered milk
avocados
boysenberries
cantaloupe
oranges
mangos
mulberries
pineapple juice
kale
turnip greens
wheat germ and bran

Top Sources of Biotin

organ meats
egg yolk
chocolate
walnuts
almonds
beef
cheese
wheat bran and germ

mushrooms
cauliflower
chicken
sardines
oysters
peanuts or peanut butter
soybean flour
rice polishings

Top Sources of Bioflavonoids

alfalfa leaf powder
apricots
buckwheat
cherries
tangerine juice
citrus pulp
citrus rind
cantaloupe
oranges
orange juice
grapefruit
grapefruit juice
broccoli

blackberries
hot red peppers
sweet red peppers
pure raw vinegar
bee propolis
plums
strawberries
elderberries
grapes
green peppers
herbal teas
red onions
black currants

Top Sources of Calcium

savory
basil
whey
marjoram, dried
thyme
dill weed
celery seed
sage
oregano
rosemary leaves
parsley, dried
(or parsley juice)
poppy seed
parmesan cheese

aged cheeses
balckstrap molasses
hazelnuts
sardines
soybean flour
turnip greens
almonds
caviar
trout
salmon
dried figs
sour cream
whole milk
yogurt

Top Sources of Iron

thyme
parsley leaves, dried
marjoram, dried
cumin seed
celery seed
dill weed, dried
oregano
bay leaves
basil
coriander leaf, dried
turmeric
cinnamon
savory
anise seed
fenugreek seed
tarragon
curry powder

liver
sardines
prunes
raisins
beef
spinach
caviar
cocoa
oysters
rice bran
soybean flour
sunflower seed flour
parsley
apricots, dried
blackstrap molasses
egg yolks
wheat bran and germ

Top Sources of Chromium

liver
brewer's yeast
blackstrap molasses
cheese

eggs
apple peels
fresh red meats

Top Sources of Copper

oysters
liver (beef, calf or lamb)
molasses, blackstrap
cocoa
black pepper
brewer's yeast
Brazil nuts
lobster
soybean flour

green olives
walnuts
almonds
wheat germ
pecans
alfalfa meal
dried coconut
lamb meat
peanut butter

Top Sources of Selenium

Brazil nuts
butter
lobster
smelt
cider vinegar
clams
crab
eggs
lamb
mushrooms

oysters
garlic
cinnamon
chili powder
nutmeg
Swiss chard
turnips
radishes
fresh whole grains

Top Sources of Magnesium

coriander leaf, dried
wheat bran and germ
dill weed
celery seed
sage
mustard, dried
basil
cocoa
fennel seed
savory
cumin seed
sesame seed flour (or paste)
tarragon

marjoram
poppy seed
Brazil nuts
rice bran
soybean flour
almonds
cashews
oat flour
whole wheat flour
beet greens
blackstrap molasses
parsley
spinach (fresh)

Top Sources of Manganese

rice bran
rice polishings
cloves
ginger
walnuts
peanuts
navy beans
lima beans
soybean flour
blackstrap molasses

blueberries
sunflower seeds
raw potatoes
lettuce
whole grains
brewer's yeast
carrots
turnips
cherries, raw
brown rice

Top Sources of Phosphorus

cocoa
pumpkin seeds
squash seeds
rice bran
rice polishings
soybean flour
sardines
mackerel
trout
herring
sunflower seeds
wheat germ

whole grain flours
red meat
almonds
egg yolks
nuts
cheese
liver
chicken
turkey
pheasant
duck

Top Sources of Zinc

oysters (raw)
sesame seed flour
 (or paste)
poppy seeds
crab
torula yeast
maple syrup
onions
wheat bran and germ
chervil, dried
cardamom
alfalfa seeds
celery seeds
basil, dried

egg yolks
lamb
popcorn
turkey (dark meat)
cheddar cheese
peanuts
peanut butter
mustard seeds, yellow
caraway seeds
egg yolks
thyme, ground
liver
beef

Top Sources of Potassium

beans
sardines
Swiss chard
veal
turkey
spinach, raw
squash (winter)
bananas
melons
orange juice
grapefruit juice
guavas
dark leafy greens
seaweed or kelp
coriander leaf, dried
parsley, dried
tomato juice
basil

dill weed, dried
tarragon
blackstrap molasses
turmeric
paprika
whey
cabbage
red pepper
soybean flour
dried apricots
dried peaches
raisins
figs
dried apples
avocados
peanuts
dates

Nutrient-Dense Foods
(Super-Rich Food Sources of Vitamins and Minerals)

rice polishings
wheat bran and germ
corn bran and germ
oat bran
brown rice
wild rice
beet and turnip tops
ground flaxseed
red hot pepper sauce
spices
pepper paste
watercress
herring
ginger
yogurt
kefir cheese
eggs
crude raw honey
avocados
salmon
herring

wild game
bison meat
homemade soups
bee pollen
fresh vegetable juices
liver (organ meats)
caraway seeds
poppy seeds
pine nuts
almonds
Brazil nuts
hazelnuts
pecans
pistachios
sunflower seeds
pumpkin or squash seeds
watermelon seeds
sesame seeds
Sesame seed paste
sardines
lecithin

Appendix B

Recipes

Thiamine Shake

3 heaping tablespoons rice polishings (or Nutri-Sense)[1]
2 to 3 tablespoons pine nuts
1 tablespoon raw sunflower seeds
1 or 2 tablespoons raw honey
8 ounces yogurt or kefir
fruit (optional)

Combine all ingredients in blender and blend until smooth. Add water to achieve desired thickness. This recipe is rich in thiamine, other B-vitamins, protein, essential fatty acids, and chromium.

Riboflavin Shake

2 tablespoons brewer's yeast
3 heaping tablespoons whey
8 ounces whole milk (goat's milk is preferable)
2 tablespoons almonds, blanched

Blend all ingredients in blender until smooth. Add water to achieve desired thickness. This recipe is rich in riboflavin, other B-vitamins, chromium, and protein. Natural strawberry flavoring enhances the taste.

Niacin Shake

3 tablespoons brewer's yeast
4 heaping tablespoons rice polishings (or Nutri-Sense)
8 to 10 ounces whole milk, water, or orange juice
1/2 cup dehydrated apricots or peaches

Blend all ingredients in blender until smooth. This recipe is rich in niacin, thiamine, riboflavin, and chromium.

---

1. *Nutri-Sense* is an excellent tasting rice polishings-based drink mix and is used as a substitute for the polishings. It offers the advantage of containing other nutrient-dense ingredients.

Pantothenic Acid Shake

1 tablespoon royal jelly
3 heaping tablespoons rice polishings (or Nutri-Sense)
8 ounces milk, juice, or water
2 tablespoons liquid pantothenic acid
2 egg whites (from farm-raised range chickens only; be sure to wash the outside before cracking)

Blend all ingredients in blender until smooth. This recipe is rich in pantothenic acid, niacin, thiamine, and chromium.

Vitamin B-6 Shake

2 heaping tablespoons rice polishings (or Nutri-Sense)
3 heaping tablespoons whey
3 tablespoons raw hazelnuts and/or sunflower seeds
1 tablespoon liquid vitamin B-6
10 ounces cold water or juice

Blend all ingredients in blender until smooth and serve chilled. This recipe is rich in vitamin B-6, other B-vitamins, vitamin E, chromium, and essential fatty acids.

Biotin Shake

2 tablespoons wheat germ
1 tablespoon cocoa powder
3 tablespoons almonds, blanched
2 heaping tablespoons rice polishings (or Nutri-Sense)
8 ounces milk
1 tablespoon honey, optional
cold water

Blend all ingredients in blender until smooth. Add cold water to adjust thickness; replace cocoa with fruit if you have a cocoa allergy. This recipe is rich in biotin, other B-vitamins, magnesium, chromium, and iron.

Folic Acid Shake

3 heaping tablespoons rice polishings (or Nutri-Sense)
1/4 cup powdered milk
4 heaping tablespoons soybean flour
1 tablespoon bee pollen
10 ounces cold water or fresh squeezed orange juice
additional cold water as needed
ripe banana or papaya (optional)

Blend all ingredients in blender to desired thickness. Add water to dilute, if necessary. This recipe is rich in protein, potassium, chromium, vitamin C, folic acid and other B-vitamins.

Folic Acid Tropical Fruit Drink

1/2 mango, peeled
1/4 cup fresh pineapple, cubed
juice of three oranges, freshly squeezed
1/2 whole avocado (optional), peeled and cubed
1 tablespoon bee pollen (optional)
6 ounces chilled coconut milk (optional)
6 to 8 ounces cold water

Add all ingredients to blender and blend until smooth. This recipe is rich in folic acid, vitamin C, and enzymes.

Folic Acid Vegetable Juice Cocktail

2 bunches parsley
4 beets, raw and peeled
1/2 head cabbage (be sure to remove tough outer leaves)
1 bunch curly endive

Wash the vegetables thoroughly under cold water. Juice in a juicer, discard pulp and serve chilled. This recipe is rich in folic acid, bioflavonoids, vitamin C, and iron.

Chromium Shake

3 or 4 heaping tablespoons rice polishings (or Nutri-Sense)
1 heaping tablespoon brewer's yeast
3 teaspoons blackstrap molasses
1 or 2 cups cow's or goat's milk
cold water

Add all ingredients in blender and blend to desired thickness, adding water to dilute, if necessary. This recipe is extremely rich in chromium as well as magnesium and B-vitamins.

Magnesium Milk Shake

4 heaping tablespoons rice polishings (or Nutri-Sense)
6 or 8 raw Brazil nuts
2 heaping tablespoons soybean flour
1 tablespoon cocoa powder
1 or 2 tablespoons raw honey
ripe banana (optional)
12 ounces milk (or cold water)
additional cold water

Add all ingredients in blender and blend until smooth, mixing additional water to reach desired thickness. This recipe is rich in magnesium, potassium, chromium, protein, niacin, and thiamine.

Magnesium-Rich Spicy Vegetable Juice Cocktail

4 tablespoons fresh dill
2 jalapeno peppers, cored, seeds removed
8 ounces Snappy Tom tomato juice cocktail, spicy V-8, or spicy Very Veggie
2 to 4 ounces cold water
1 teaspoon celery seed
bunch of watercress or parsley (optional)

Blend all ingredients in blender until smooth and serve chilled. For extra flavor juice watercress or parsley and add to the drink. This recipe is rich in magnesium, potassium, beta carotene, and vitamin C.

Potassium-Rich Vegetable Juice Cocktail

2 cups fresh coriander leaves (cilantro)
1 bunch parsley
1 head romaine lettuce
1/2 cup chopped red sweet peppers
1 carrot, peeled, optional (for additional sweetness)

Add all ingredients to juice extractor; serve chilled. This recipe is rich in magnesium, potassium, vitamin C, and beta carotene.

Enzymatic Fruit-Sweetened Milk Shake

1 or 2 tablespoon(s) raw bee pollen
1/4 cup strawberries or blueberries
1/4 cup diced fresh pineapple
8 ounces fresh raw milk (goat's milk preferred)
2 tablespoons rice polishings (or Nutri-Sense)
1 or 2 tablespoons pure raw honey
cold water

Add all ingredients to blender and blend until smooth, mixing additional water to desired thickness. Drink immediately. This recipe is rich in enzymes, vitamin C, magnesium, and B-vitamins.

Enzymatic Fruit Splash

3 ripe pomegranates, seeds removed
3 kiwis, peeled
1 large papaya, peeled
1 mango, peeled (optional)
2 or 4 ounces cold-processed aloe vera liquid
cold water

Blend in blender until smooth, adding water to achieve desired thickness. This recipe is rich in enzymes, folic acid, and vitamin C.

Protein/Amino Acid Shake

3 tablespoons soybean flour
1/4 cup powdered milk
1/4 cup sunflower seeds
2 tablespoons bee pollen
12 ounces cold water (or milk)

Add all ingredients to blender and blend until well-mixed, adding extra water if necessary. This recipe is rich in amino acids, B-vitamins, potassium, copper, and vitamin E.

Sea Salt/Sodium Tomato Juice Cocktail

2 teaspoons sea salt, (preferably Celtic salt)
6 ounces tomato juice (unsalted)
juice of three or four ripe tomatoes
Tabasco sauce (optional)
cold water
1 tablespoon capers

Blend all ingredients in blender except capers; add water to achieve desired thickness. Serve chilled or over ice. This recipe is rich in sodium, other trace minerals, and vitamin C.

Gingerized Liver Regeneration Drink

1 medium raw ginger root, peeled
1 cup black radish (or daikon radish), peeled and cubed
1 bunch watercress, carefully washed in cold water
1 head romaine lettuce, carefully washed in cold water
1 avocado, peeled (as a source of fat to stimulate bile flow)
cold water

Juice the ginger and vegetables; discard pulp. In a blender add juice and avocado and blend until well mixed; add cold water as needed to achieve desired consistency. This recipe is rich in bioflavonoids, vitamin C, potassium, and vitamin K.

Vitamin C-Fortified Fruit Cocktail

1/4 cup strawberries, preferably fresh and pesticide-free
2 kiwi fruits, peeled
10 ounces fresh squeezed organic grapefruit or orange juice
1/2 teaspoon powdered vitamin C

Blend all ingredients in blender until smooth. This recipe is rich in vitamin C and bioflavonoids.

Vitamin K Vegetable Juice Cocktail

1 bunch spinach or watercress
3 tablespoons powdered alfalfa leaves (not the seeds; they are toxic)
2 cups chopped beet greens (wash well)
1/2 head green cabbage, outer leaves removed

Add all ingredients to a juice extractor. Serve chilled. This recipe is rich in vitamin K, vitamin C, bioflavonoids, and calcium.

Calcium-Rich Vegetable Juice Cocktail

1 cup carrot juice
2 bunches watercress, carefully washed in cold water
1 bunch romaine lettuce, carefully washed in cold water
1 bunch parsley
2 teaspoons of powdered calcium supplement or calcium ascorbate
cold water

Blend all ingredients in blender, adding water to achieve desired thickness, and serve chilled.

Anti-Aging Vegetable Juice Cocktail

3 medium or large carrots, washed and peeled
1 bunch watercress, carefully washed in cold water
4 turnips, washed and peeled
8 radishes (include tops if fresh—wash thoroughly)
2 ounces aloe vera juice (optional)
1 head romaine lettuce (wash leaves thoroughly)

Blend all ingredients in blender, adding water to achieve desired thickness, and serve chilled.

Appendix C

Ordering Information for
Books and Nutritional Products

Address for Ordering

All of the unique nutritional products mentioned in this book and listed below may be ordered from:

NUTRITIONAL SUPPLEMENT SERVICE
212 Willow Parkway
Buffalo Grove, Illinois 60089
(800) 243-5242

Nutritional/Health Products

Fat-Soluble Thiamine
Anti-Aging Vitamin Cream
Balancing Infusion
Premium-Grade Vitamin E
Premium-Grade Selenium
Premium-Grade Pycnogenol
Premium-Grade Beta Carotene
Premium-Grade Aloe Vera Extract
Iron-Free Multi-Vitamin/Mineral
Water Filtration Straw
Potassium Gluconate
Pharmaceutical-Grade Chelated Zinc
Progest Cream and Sublingual Drops
Emulsified Oil of Oregano
Detergent-Free Vitamin A Drops
Nutri-Sense Protein Drink Mix

Organic Silica
Zinc Tally
N-Acetyl Cysteine
Glutathione
Livit-2
Lipoic Acid
Megadose Biotin
Tanalbit
Intestinalis
Magnesium Taurate
Formula 416
Ground Flax Seed
Dessicated Buffalo Liver
Mexican Yam Extract
Organic Iodine Drops
Rice Polishings

Specialty Food Products

Hawaiian Shark Jerky (excellent source of
  shark cartilage and unprocessed protein)
  Other jerky products available soon
Premium-Grade Imported Bee Propolis,
  Pollen, and Honey Mixture (excellent
  for internal and/or topical use)

To order call
800-98SHARK

800-658-4406

Price-Pottenger Nutrition Foundation

This non-profit foundation offers a newsletter and health care provider referral service. The referral service provides the individual with lists by state for locating nutritionally oriented doctors/practitioners. In addition, a number of invaluable nutritional books are available from the Price-Pottenger Nutrition Foundation. A sampling of these books includes:

Nutrition and Physical Degeneration
by Weston Price, D.D.S.
Pottenger's Cats: A study in nutrition
by F.M. Pottenger Jr., M.D.
Your Family Tree Connection
by Chris Reading, M.D.
Degeneration-Regeneration
by Melvin Page, D.D.S.
Enzyme Nutrition
by Edward Howell
For Tomorrow's Children: A Manual for Future Parents
by Pre-Conception Care, Inc.
Candida Albicans Yeast-Free Cookbook
by Pat Connoly
The Get Healthy Cookbook
by Bessie Joe Tillman, M.D.
Root Canal Cover-up Exposed
by George E. Meinig, D.D.S.

The Price-Pottenger Foundation produces a quarterly newsletter/journal. It is packed with invaluable information about the latest findings in the fields of nutrition, preventive medicine, ecology, recipe creation, and organic gardening. Articles by Dr. Igram, who is an advisory board member, are featured in the journal. Address inquiries to the Price-Pottenger Nutrition Foundation, 2667 Camino Del Rio South, #109, San Diego, CA 92108, or call 1-800-Foods-4-U (1-800-366-3748).

Bibliography

Abraham, A.S., et al. 1987. Magnesium in the prevention of lethal arrhythmias in acute myocardial infarction. *Arch. Intern. Med.* 147:753.

Adams, P.W., et al. 1973. Effect of pyridoxine hydrochloride (vitamin B-6) upon depression associated with oral contraception. *The Lancet* 1:899.

Coggeshall, J.C., Heggers, J.P., Robson, M.C., et al. 1985. Biotin status and plasma glucose in diabetics. *Annal. N.Y. Acad. Sci.* 447:389.

Collip, P.J., et al. 1975. Pyridoxine treatment of childhood bronchial asthma. *Ann. Allergy.* 35:93.

Collins, E.B., and P. Ardt. 1980. Inhibition of C. Albicans by lactobacilli and lactobacillic fermented dairy products. *FEMS Micro. Rev.* (Sept.), 46:343.

Cook, J.D., et al. 1974. Serum ferritin as a measure of iron in normal subjects. *Amer. J. Clin. Nutr.* 27:9681-87.

Cragin, R.B. 1962. The use of bioflavonoids in the prevention and treatment of athletic injuries. *Med. Times* 90:529.

Crittinden, P.J. 1948. Studies on the pharmacology of biotin. *Arch. Int. Pharm. Ther.* 76:263.

Curtis, A.C., and R.S. Baliner. 1939. The prevention of carotene absorption by liquid petrolatum. *JAMA* 113:1785.

Dakashinamurti, K., and H.N. Bhagavan (eds). 1985. *Biotin.* New York: The New York Academy of Science.

Davis, Adelle. 1965. *Let's Get Well.* New York: Signet.

Davies, S., and A. Stewart. 1987. *Nutritional Medicine.* London: Pan Books.

Dean, R., and K. Cheesman. 1987. Vitamin E protects against free radical damage in lipid environment *Bioc. Biop. R.* 148:1277-82.

DiLuzio, N.R. 1973. Antioxidants, lipid peroxidation, and chemical-induced liver injury. *Fed. Proc.* 32:1875-81.

Diplock, A.T. 1980. The role of vitamin E and selenium in the prevention of oxygen-induced tissue damage. In. Selenium in Biology and Medicine, *Proceedings Second International Symposium.* Westport, CT: AVI Publ.

Drake, M.E. 1986. Panic attacks and excessive aspartamine ingestion. *The Lancet* 2:631.

Editor. 1992. Neurologic signs of B-12 deficiency. *Emergency Med.* July, pp. 198-202.

Editors. 1984. *The Complete Book of Vitamins.* Emmaus, PA: Rodale Press.

Ensminger, A.H., et al. 1983. *Foods and Nutrition Encyclopedia.* Vol. 1&2. Clovis, CA: Pergus Press.

Erasmus, U. 1989. *Fats and Oils.* Burnaby, BC: Alive Books.

Fernandes, K.M., and M.A. Shahani. 1987. Therapeutic role of dietary lactobacilli and lactobacillic fermented dairy products. *FEMS Micro. Rev.* 46:343.

Florence, T.M. 1984. Cancer and aging: the free radical connection. Int. *Clin. Nutr. Rev.* 4(1), pp. 6-19.

Folkers, K., and Y. Yamamura (eds). 1986. *Biomedical and Clinical Applications of Coenzyme Q-10.* Bantam Books.

Freedman, A., et al. 1990. Magnesium deficiency-induced cardiomyopathy: protection by vitamin E. *Bioc. Biop. Res. Comm.* 170:1102.

Frolkis, V.V., et al. 1987. Antioxidants as antiarrhythmic drugs. *Cardiology* 74:124.

Frost, D.V, and P.M. Lish. 1975. Selenium in biology. *Ann. Rev. Pharm.* 75:259-84.

Fujisawa, K., Suzuki, H., et al. 1984. Therapeutic effects of liver hydrolysate preparation on chronic hepatitis—a double blind, controlled study. *Asian Med. J.* 26:497-526.

Gabor, M. 1972. Pharmacologic effect of flavonoids on blood vessels. *Angiologica* 9:355.

Gallagher, J.C., et al. 1979. Intestinal calcium absorption and serum vitamin D metabolites in normal subjects and osteoporotic patients. *J. Clin. Invest.* 64:729.

Gibson, G.E., et al. 1988. Reduced activities of thiamine-dependent enzymes in the brains and peripheral tissue of patients with Alzheimer's disease. *Arch. Neuro.* 45:836-40.

Gilliland, S.E., and M.K. Speck. 1977. Antagonistic action of Lactobacillus acidophilus toward intestinal and food-borne pathogens in associative cultures. *J. Food Product.* 40:830.

Gloor, M., and H. Fischer. 1971. Principles of flavonoid therapy. *Fortschr. Med.* 89:1025.

Goldberg, I.K. 1980. L-tyrosine in depression. *The Lancet* 2:364.

311

Goldman, I.S., and N.E. Kantrowitz. 1982. Cardiomyopathy associated with selenium deficiency. *NEJM* 305:701.

Green, H.N., and E. Mellanby. 1928. Vitamin A as an anti-infective agent. *Br. Med. J.* 20:691.

Greenwood, J. 1965. Optimal vitamin C intake as a factor in the preservation of disc integrity. *Med. Ann. Distr.* Col. 33:274.

Hackney, J.D., et al. 1975. Experimental studies on human health effects of air pollutants. II Ozone. *Arch. Envir. Hlth.* 30:379-84.

Halliwell, B., and J.M.C. Gutteridge. 1984. Lipid peroxidation, oxygen radicals, cell damage, and antioxidant therapy. *The Lancet*, pp. 1396.

Hammar, M., Larson, L, and L. Tegler. 1981. Calcium treatment of leg cramps in pregnancy. *Acta. Obstet. Gynecol. Scand.* 60:345-47.

Haun, R.J. 1992. Indicators of poor nutritional status in older Americans. *Amer. Fam. Phys.* Jan, pp. 219-27.

Havsteen, B. 1983. Flavonoids, a class of natural products of high pharmacological potency. *Biochem. Pharm.* 32:1141.

Heimburger, D., et al. 1987. Improvement in bronchial squamous metaplasia in smoker treated with folate and B-12. *Amer. J. Clin. Nutr.* 45:866.

Hill, M.J., Drasar, B.S., Aries, V., et al. 1971. Bacteria and the etiology of cancer of the large bowel. *The Lancet* 1:95-100.

Hingerty, D. 1957. The role of magnesium in adrenal insufficiency. *Biochem. J.* 66:429-31.

Horrobin, D.F., and M.S. Manku. 1983. Essential fatty acids in clinical medicine. *Nutrition and Health* 2:127-34.

Horwitt, M.K. 1980. Relative biological values of D-alpha-tocopheryl acietate and all-rac-A tocopheryl acetate in man. *Amer. J. Clin. Nutr.* 33:1856.

Horwitt, M.K. 1980. Therapeutic use of vitamin E in medicine. *Nutr. Rev.* 38(3).

Igram, Cass. 1989. *Eat Right to Live Long*. Cedar Rapids, IA: Literary Visions.

Igram, Cass. 1990. *Who Needs Headaches?* Cedar Rapids, IA: Literary Visions.

Iseri, L.T., et al. 1975. Magnesium deficiency and cardiac disorders. *Amer. J. Med.* 58:837.

Ishiyama, T., et al. 1976. A clinical study of the effect of coenzyme Q on congestive heart failure. *Japan Heart J.* 17:32.

Isselbacher, K.J. 1977. Metabolic and hepatic effect of alcohol. *NEJM* (Mar), 296(11).

Jacobsen, H.N., et al (eds). 1983. *Manual of Clinical Nutrition.* Pleasantville, NJ: Nutrition Publications, Inc.

Johns, D.R. 1986. Migraine provoked by aspartame. *NEJM.*

Johnson, F.C. 1979. The antioxidant vitamins. *CRC Crit. Rev. Food Sci. Nutr.* 11:217-309.

Kamm, J.J., Dashman, T., Newark, H., et al. 1977. Inhibition of amine nitrite hepatotoxicity by alpha-tocopherol. *Toxicol. Appl. Pharm.* 41:575-83.

Karkkainen, P., et al. 1986. Alcohol intake correlated with serum trace elements. *Alc. Alcohol* 23:279-82.

Kaul, T.N., Middleton, E., and P.L. Ogra. 1985. Anti-viral effect of flavonoids on human viruses. *J. Med. Virol.* 15:71-9.

Khan, A., et. al. 1990. Insulin potentiating factor and chromium content of selected foods and spices. *Biol. Tr. Elem. Res.* 24:183.

Kligman, A., et al. 1981. Oral vitamin A in acne vulgaris. *Int. J. Derm.* 20:278.

Kok, F.J., et al. 1986. Dietary sodium, calcium, and potassium, and blood pressure. *Amer. J. Epid.* 123:1043-48.

Kolata, G. 1982. Heart study produces a surprise result. *Science* 218:31-2.

Kondoh, M., et al. 1984. Effect of sodium saccharin on rate pancreatic enzyme secretion. *J. Nutr. Sci. Vitam.* 30:569.

Krause, M.V., and L.K. Mahan. 1984. *Food, Nutrition, and Diet Therapy.* Philadelphia: W.B. Saunders Co.

Krinsky, N., et al. 1982. Interaction of oxygen and oxy-radicals with carotenoids. *J. Can. Res. Clin. Onco.* 69:205.

Kromhout, D. 1992. Dietary fatty acids, serum cholesterol, and 25-year mortality from coronary heart disease: The Seven Countries Study. *Circulation* 85:864.

Lawson, M., et al. 1987. The effect of dietary fibre on apparent absorption of zinc, copper, iron and manganese in the elderly. *P. Nutr. Soc.* 46:53A.

LeGrady, D., et al. 1987. Coffee consumption and mortality in the Chicago Western Electric Company. *Am. J. Epid.* 126:803.

Lesser, M. 1980. *Nutrition and Vitamin Therapy.* New York: Bantam.

Leonart, M.S.S. 1989. Effect of vitamin E on red blood cell preservation. Braz. *J. Med. Biol. Res.* 22:85-6.

Lindenbaum, J., et al. 1988. Neuropsychiatric disorders caused by cobalamin deficiency in the absence of anemia or macrocytosis. *NEJM* 318:1720-28.

Littarru, G.P., Ho, L., and K. Folkers. 1972. Deficiency of coenzyme Q-10 in human heart disease. II. *Internat. J. Vit. Res.* 42:413.

Lonsdale, D. 1987. Thiamine and its fat soluble derivatives as therapeutic agents. *Int. Clin. Nutr. Rev.* 1(3):114-25.

Manson, J., et al. 1992. A prospective study of vitamin C and incidence of coronary heart disease in women. *Circulation* 85:865.

Massey, L., et al. 1988. Acute effects of dietary caffeine and aspirin on urinary mineral excretion in pre- and postmenopausal women. *Nutr. Res.* pp. 845-51.

Matz, R. 1993. Magnesium Deficiencies and Therapeutic Uses. *Hospital Practice.* Apr 30.

McClain, C.J., and L. Su. 1983. Zinc deficiency in the alcoholic: a review. *Alcoholism: Clin. and Exper. Res.* 7(1).

Middleton, E. 1984. The flavonoids, trends in pharmaceutical science. *Science* 5:335.

Mock, D., Johnson, S., and R. Holman. 1988. Effects of biotin deficiency on serum fatty acid composition: evidence for abnormalities in humans. *J. Nutr.* 118:342.

Moses, H.A. 1979. Trace elements: an association with cardiovascular diseases and hypertension. *J. Natl Med. Assoc.* 71:227-28.

Mussalo-Rauhamma, H., et al. 1987. Decreased serum selenium and magnesium levels in drunkeness arrestees. *Drug Alc. Dep.* 20:95.

Niki, E., Tsuchiya, J. Yoshikawa, Y., et al. 1986. Oxidation of lipids. XIII. Anti oxidant activites of alpha-, beta-, gamma-, and delta-tocopherols. *Bull. Chem. Soc. Jpn.* 59:497-501.

Oelgetz, A.W., et al. 1935. The treatment of food allergy and indigestion of pancreatic origin with pancreatic enzymes. *Amer. J. Dig. Dis. Nutr.* 2:422-426.

Oelgetz, A.W., et al. 1939. Pancreatic enzymes and food allergy. *Med. Rec.* 150:276-279.

Paris, R., and J. Moury. 1964. Effects of diverse flavonoids upon capillary permeability. *Ann. Pharm. Frac.* 22:489-923.

Perry, H.M. 1978. *Effect of Nutrient Deficiencies in Man: Selenium in Handbook Series in Nutrition and Food*, Sect. E., Vol. III, M. Rechcigl ed., CRC Press.

Peticone, F., et al. 1988. Protective magnesium treatment in ischemic dilated cardiomyopathy (meeting abstract). *J. Am. Col. Nutr.* 7:403.

Prasad, K.N. 1983. Effects of tocopherol on morhological alterations and growth inhibition in melanoma cells in culture. *Cancer Res.* 42:550.

Prasad, K.N. 1984. Nutrition and cancer. In *Yearbook of Nutritional Medicine.* J. Bland. (ed). 1:178-189.

Raloff, J. 1986. Reasons for boning up on maganese. *Science News* (Sept.) 130:199.

Randi, A., et al. 1987. Orally administered vitamin B-6 prolongs the bleeding time and inhibits platelet aggregation in human volunteers. *Thromb. Haem.* 58:176.

Rasad, A.S. 1981. Zinc in growth and development and spectrum of human zinc life. *T.A.M. Coll. Nutr.* 7:377.

Reed, I.J. 1953. Metabolic functions of thiamin and lipoic acid. *Physical Rev.* 33:544-559.

Reid, I.R., and H.K. Ibbertson. 1986. Calcium supplements in the prevention of steriod-induced osteoporosis. *Amer. J. Clin. Nutr.* 44:287-290.

Reiser, S., et al. 1987. Effect of copper intake on blood cholesterol and its lipoprotein distribution in men. *Nutr. Rep. In.* 36:641-649.

Resnik, L. 1987. Interrelation of calcium and magnesium with renin-sodium factors in essential hypertension. *J. Am. Coll. Nutr.* 6:62-63.

Reynolds, E., et al. 1971. Folate metabolism in epileptic and psychiatric patients. *J. Neuro. Neurosurg. Psych.* 34:726.

Riales, R. and M. Albrink. 1981. Effects of chronium chloride supplementation on the glucose tolerance and serum lipids, including HDL, in adult men. *Am. J. Clin. Nutr.* 34:2670-2678.

Rice, S.L., Eiten Miller, R.R., Koehler, P.E. 1976. Biologically active amines in food: a review. *J. Milk. Food Techno.* 39(5):353-358.

Roe, D.A. 1983. *Drug-Induced Nutritional Deficiencies.* A.V.I., Westport, CN.

Roe, D.A. 1986. Nutritional Assessment of the elderly. *Wld. Rev. Nutr. Diet.* 48:85-113.

Rogers, S. 1985. Sugar and health. *The Lancet* Feb. 23.

Rosenberg, E., and P. Belew. 1982. Microbial factors in psoriasis. *Arch. Derm.* 118:1434-1444.

Sandine, W.E. 1979. Roles of lactobacillus in test intestinal tract. *Journal of Food Protection* 42:259-262.

Scholar, E., et al. 1988. Effects of diets enriched in cabbage and collards on metastasis of BALB/c mammary carcinoma (meeting abstract). *P. Am. Assoc. Ca.* 29:149.

Schrauzer, G.N. (ed.). 1988. *Selenium, in Biological Trace Element Research.* Humana Press.

Schrauzer, G.N. and D.A. White. 1978. Selenium in human nutrition: dietary intakes and effects of supplementation. *Bioinorganic Chemistry* 8:303-318.

Schrauzer, G.N. 1977 Cancer mortalitiy correlation studies III. Statistical associations with dietary selenium intakes. *Bioinorganic Chemistry* 7:23.

Schrauzer, G.N. 1976. Selenium and cancer: a review. *Bioinorganic Chemistry* 5:275.

Schroeder, H.A. 1973. *The Trace Elements and Man.* Devin-Adair Co., Old Greenwich, CN.

Schroeder, H.A. 1974. *The Poisons Around Us.* Indiana Univ. Press, London.

Seelig, M. 1964. The requirement of magnesium by the normal adult. *Amer. J. Clin. Nutr.* 14:242-290.

Shamberger, R.J. 1976. *Selenium in health and disease. Proc. Symp. Selen. Tell. Envir.* Industrial Health Foundation, Inc., Pittsburg, PA.

Shariff, R., et al. 1988. Vitamin E supplementation in smokers. *Clin. Res.* 36:A770.

Shaw, D.M., et al. 1984. Senile dementia and nutrition (letter to the editor). *Brit. Med. J.* 288:792-793.

Sohler, A, Kruesi, M., Pfeiffer, C2C2 1977. Blood lead levels in psychiatric outpatients reduced by zinc and vitamin C. *J. Orthomol. Psy.* 6(3):272-276.

Sommer, A. 1990. Vitamin A status, resistance to infection,and childhood mortality. *Ann. NY Acad. Sci.* 587:17.

Stauber, P., et al. 1991. A longitudinal study of the relationship between vitamin A supplementation and plasma retinol, retinyl esters, and liver enzyme activities in a healthy elderly population. *Am. J. Clin. Nutr.* 54:878-883.

316

Stevens, R., et al. 1988. Body iron stores and the risk of cancer. *Am. J. Clin. Nutr.* 319:1047-1052.

Suda, D., et al. 1986. Inhibition of experimental oral carcinogensis by topical beta carotene. *Carcinogenesis* 7:711.

Sugiyama, S., Kitazawa, M., Ozawa, K., et al. 1980. Anitoxidative effect of coenzyme Q-10. *Experiontia* 36:1002.

Sullivan, J.I. 1981. Iron and the sex difference in heart disease risk. *The Lancet* June 13, p. 1239.

Sullivan, J.I. 1983. Vegetarianism, ischemic heart disease, and iron (letter to the editor). *Am. J. Clin. Nutr.* 37:882-886.

Swain, A., Dutton, S.P., Truswell, A.S. 1985. Salicylates in foods. *J. Amer. Diet. Assoc.* 85(8):950-960.

Tanaka, K. 1981. New light on biotin deficiency. *N.E.J.M.* 304:839-840.

Tappel, A.L. 1973. Lipid peroxidation damage to cell components. *Fed. Proc.* 32:1870-1874.

Index

132, 143, 148, 164, 172, 204, 246, 253; ravenous or excessive, 25, 31, 246, 269

Are You Aging Quiz, 238-244

Arthritis, 7, 14, 17, 35, 37, 42, 44, 49, 73, 45, 79, 81, 83, 87, 88, 98, 106, 107, 113, 115, 119-121, 124, 128, 130, 131, 134, 137, 138, 140, 159, 169, 172, 184, 191, 203, 206-208, 222, 231, 268, 282, 283

Aspirin, 6, 45, 50, 53, 54, 62, 64, 66, 67, 74, 78, 96, 98, 115, 117, 122, 132, 161, 172, 219

Asthma, 6, 45, 50, 53, 54, 62, 64, 66, 67, 74, 78, 90, 96, 98, 110, 115, 117, 122, 132, 161, 172, 203, 219, 225-227

Asthmatics. *See* Asthma

Atherosclerosis, 51, 79, 93, 120, 130, 182; *see also* Hardening of the arteries

Atrial fibrillation, 130

Attention deficit disorder, 25, 47, 97, 170, 172, 219, 222, 260, 264

Autism, 45, 170, 219

B

B-vitamins, 3, 5, 12, 13, 20, 22, 28, 29, 33, 34, 37, 39, 42-46, 48, 49, 52, 54, 55, 57, 58, 67, 116, 158, 165, 173, 174, 188, 193, 201, 212, 213, 223-225, 227, 228, 231, 234-236, 242, 250-251, 255-258, 261, 262, 265-267, 273, 274, 284, 285, 288

Bacteria. *See* Intestinal Bacteria

Bad breath, 35, 47

Bed sores, 78, 146

Bed wetting, 26

Bee pollen, 41, 157, 158

Beriberi, 4, 5, 7, 22, 28, 287

Beta carotene, 6, 12, 13, 67, 76, 79, 80, 188, 192, 223, 224, 229-231, 242, 243, 266, 267, 279, 280, 286; *see also* Vitamin A

Bifidus (Bifidobacteria), 175, 177, 279, 280

Bioflavonoids, 96, 158-162, 187, 229, 251, 258; top sources, 158-161

Biotin, 11, 22, 58-61, 87, 261, 262, 266, 267, 276, 279, 280; foods rich in, 59

Birth control pills, 29, 32, 45, 47, 53, 56, 64, 74, 79, 95, 150, 151, 261, 272, 278

Bladder, 12, 17, 118, 172, 228, 264, 265; cancer of, 12, 228; loss of control of, 118

Black walnut extract, 268

Bleeding disorders, 89, 161; *see also* Gums, bleeding

Blindness, 12, 77, 80; *see also* Macular degeneration

Blood clotting, 83, 89, 94, 125, 161, 278

Blood clots, 92, 160

Blood sugar, 38, 59, 60, 102, 103, 124, 131, 148, 196, 208, 215, 251, 252, 256, 258-262, 277, 282; *see also* Hypoglycemia

Blood Sugar Collapse Syndrome, 258-262

Bloodshot eyes, 30

Body odor, 118

Bone loss, 95, 97, 99; *see also* Osteoporosis

Bone pain, 85, 124, 128, 129

Bone spurs, 55

Brain, 5, 24, 28, 49, 55, 113, 116, 118, 120, 166, 170, 224, 232, 259, 264, 289

Breast cancer, 272

Bronchitis, 110, 111, 159, 203, 216
Brown spots, 92, 187
Bruises, 146, 241, 246
Bruising tendency, 73, 85, 92, 95, 158, 159, 161, 171, 176, 246
Bruxism, 41, 85
Bulimia, 26, 117
Bursitis, 41, 55

C
Caffeine, 18, 42, 54, 71, 75, 119, 203, 215, 232-236, 239, 249, 255-257, 273
Caffeine & Caffeine-Like Substance Quiz, 232-237
Calcium, 3, 12, 14, 38, 67, 83, 84, 86, 97-102, 126, 128, 138, 150, 204, 207, 224, 243; foods rich in, 100, 117
Cancer, 6-10, 12, 17, 19, 50-52, 54, 65, 67, 75, 79, 83, 86-89, 101, 105, 113, 117, 133, 134, 136-138, 140, 159, 163, 164, 170, 176, 184, 191, 196, 203, 207, 208, 219, 228-231, 235, 242, 272, 274, 276
Cancer belt, 137
Candida, 175; *see also* Fungal infection, Yeast infection, Yeast/ Fungus Syndrome
Candidiasis. *See* Candida albicans, Yeast/Fungus Syndrome
Canker sores, 52, 149
Carbohydrates, 42, 255, 261, 264
Carnitine, 257, 258, 261, 262
Carpal tunnel syndrome, 44, 45, 48, 58, 119, 247
Carotene. *See* Beta Carotene
Cataracts, 9, 32, 51, 84, 85, 89, 92, 104, 105, 137, 242
Cavities, 100, 128, 282
Celiac disease, 52, 86, 96, 106,

186, 130, 153, 283
Chapped lips, 31, 47, 52, 59, 149, 171, 179
Chemotherapy, 8, 53, 93, 100, 105, 277, 283
Chewing tobacco, 31, 53, 64, 122, 164, 230, 244
Chlorella, 57, 155, 157-158, 280, 284
Chlorinated water, 23, 27, 92, 95, 175, 177, 178, 269
Chlorine, 12, 23, 175, 177, 178, 268
Cholesterol, 9, 11, 31, 32, 34, 35, 37, 47, 60, 78, 81-83, 86, 92, 95, 96, 103, 107, 111, 123, 125, 145, 160, 170, 173, 176, 184-185, 196, 208, 239, 247, 251, 254, 273, 277, 278
Choline, 224, 234-236, 274, 276, 279, 280
Chromium, 11, 42, 102-105, 212, 213, 243, 251, 256, 257, 261, 262, 266, 287; foods rich in, 102, 103
Chronic Fatigue Syndrome, 18, 281
Cigarette smoke. *See* Cigarette smoking
Cigarette smoking, 19, 31, 50, 52, 53, 62, 64-66, 70, 71, 74, 75, 89, 91, 100, 101, 122, 162, 164, 168, 172, 229-231, 239-242, 244, 247, 253-254, 257, 264, 269
Cirrhosis, 24, 101, 105, 125, 159, 268, 275, 277
Cobalt, 15, 55
Cobalamin. *See* Vitamin B-12
Cocoa, 18, 23, 42, 114, 118, 186, 214, 232-234, 255, 257
Coenzyme Q-10, 109, 165-169, 212, 242-244, 256, 258

Constipation, 20, 25, 40, 46, 51, 55, 115, 118, 131, 152, 163, 176, 179, 193, 235, 246, 252, 264, 277, 282

Copper, 14, 15, 105-107, 109, 116, 147, 150-151, 174, 248-250, 287; foods rich in, 106

Corneal ulcers, 32, 80

Coronary artery disease, 104, 116, 122, 128, 130, 137, 168-169

Cortisone, 3, 41, 45, 47, 56, 62, 64, 74, 82, 94, 98, 100, 101, 117, 128, 129, 132, 147, 150, 173, 251, 254, 258, 261, 263, 265; *see also* Drugs

Cowlicks, 59

Crohn's disease, 50, 56, 79, 95, 117, 122, 130, 147, 153, 169, 172, 177, 265, 282, 283

D

Dandruff, 31, 59, 264, 282

Deep Fried Food Quiz, 191-193

Dehydration. *See* Water Deficiency (Dehydraton) Quiz

Delirium tremens, 29

Dementia, 5, 28, 35, 37, 83, 121, 172

Depression, 5, 7, 13, 22, 24-26, 28, 30, 35, 36, 40, 44, 46-52, 55, 59, 74, 103, 105, 114, 116, 118, 121, 131, 152, 156, 170, 208, 215, 219, 223, 224, 235, 246, 253-256, 259-260, 289

Dermatitis, 32, 35, 46, 59, 60, 136, 139, 148, 152, 169, 176, 283

Diabetic neuropathy, 45

Diabetic ulcers, 78

Diabetes, 7, 17, 28, 37, 41, 42, 44, 48, 60, 75, 79, 83, 103, 105, 107, 130, 134, 137, 153, 163,

164, 169, 184, 191, 204, 206-208, 215, 228, 231, 258-260, 262, 275, 278

Diarrhea, 14, 35, 51, 78, 85, 95, 106, 119, 120, 132, 144, 164, 171, 176, 200, 204, 252, 264, 268, 269, 282

Diseases. *See* individual entries

Dizziness, 30, 114, 118, 144, 259

Drugs, 4, 6, 8, 17, 34, 45, 50, 54, 65, 74, 78, 86, 94, 96, 98, 99, 115, 117, 132, 133, 136, 147, 151, 153, 158, 161, 162, 172, 218, 220, 233, 242, 263, 274, 276-280, 289

E

Eczema, 3, 33, 40, 41, 48, 81, 85, 136, 139, 140, 160, 164, 169, 171, 176, 203, 242, 264, 283

Edema, 49, 131, 227; *see also* Fluid retention

Electrolytes, 178, 142

Emphysema, 65, 75, 79, 93, 110, 168, 172

Endocrine system, 255

Endometriosis, 153, 233, 234, 265, 272

Enzymes, 2, 12, 13, 15, 16, 58, 76, 106, 109, 123, 147, 154, 157, 158, 162-169, 208, 242, 244, 276, 278, 281, 284, 286

Epilepsy, 45, 46, 48, 49, 86, 120

Essential fatty acids, 43, 59, 169-174, 178, 180, 188, 192, 224, 286; deficiency of, 170, 178, 286; foods rich in, 169, 170, 171, 173; gamma linolenic acid (GLA), 174

Estrogen, 82, 83, 252, 271-175

Eyes, 30-33, 47, 51, 55, 74, 78, 132, 149, 172, 179, 238-240,

247, 269, 277; dryness of, 47, 78, 172, 179, 240, 269

F

Fatigue, 5, 13, 25, 31, 35, 36, 38, 39, 42, 46, 52, 55, 65, 66, 73, 88, 103, 106, 111, 114, 118, 128, 131, 143, 152, 156, 164, 167, 204, 208, 212, 119, 225, 235, 240, 250-252, 259, 269, 277, 282, 289, 290; *see also* Chronic fatigue syndrome

Fatty acids, 11, 16, 43, 59, 127, 169-171, 173, 174, 178, 180, 188, 192, 224, 251, 286; *see also* Essential fatty acids

Fainting spells, 40, 132, 252, 259

Fiber, 193, 196, 198

Fibrocystic breast disease, 89, 93, 172, 233, 234, 272

Fibromyalgia, 17, 49, 160

Fibromyositis, 17, 49, 140, 153

Fingernails, 115, 146, 148, 164, 171, 240, 246, 264, 278

Fish oils, 170

Flu, 201, 212, 216, 219, 223, 225, 241, 268

Fluid retention, 44, 46, 145

Folic Acid, 11, 12, 49-54, 58, 109, 152, 153, 224, 227, 228, 231, 236, 267, 273, 274, 281, 284, 285, 287; foods rich in, 11, 51, 53

Folic Acid Shake, 54, 303

Food allergies, 40, 147, 198, 203, 253, 281, 283-286

Food Dye Quiz, 216-219

Fungal infections, 111, 136, 137, 212, 254, 262-264, 268, 270, 271, 278; *see also* Candida albicans, Yeast infection, Yeast/ Fungus Syndrome

G

Garlic, 135, 192, 229-231, 243-245, 266, 280

Geographic tongue, 148, 282

Genetic defects, 5, 204

Giardiasis, 24, 147, 268, 278

Gilbert's disease, 24, 275

Ginger, 125, 130, 159, 268, 271, 274, 289, 290, 284

Glutathione, 187, 188, 192, 213, 224, 229-231, 242, 244, 276

Goiter, 108, 110, 111, 245

Goitrogens, 112, 249

Gout, 41, 50, 53, 125, 149

Gum disease, 52, 79, 128, 166, 167

Gums, bleeding, 52, 73, 95, 159, 160, 167, 171

H

Hair, 14, 32, 40, 41, 46, 47, 52, 56, 58, 59, 77, 78, 106, 111, 114, 115, 130, 136, 139, 140, 147-149, 152-154, 156, 164, 171, 240, 246, 247, 254, 273, 276, 282; brittle, 47, 52, 59, 77, 114, 139, 148, 156, 171, 247; loss of, 14, 40, 47, 59, 60, 106, 115, 136, 139, 148, 152, 154, 156, 164, 169, 171, 240, 246, 253, 277, 282; premature graying of, 41, 56, 140, 149, 152, 153, 238, 240, 282

Hardening of the arteries, 6, 60, 74, 93, 104, 104, 107, 116, 132, 170, 184, 206, 242, 247

Headaches, 5-7, 12, 26, 35, 40, 49, 66, 100, 114, 119, 132, 143, 152, 170, 201, 203, 212, 219, 223, 225-227, 231, 234, 235, 246, 247, 252, 260, 261, 273, 283, 289

Heart disease, 6, 7, 9, 10, 17, 19,

also Acidophilus, Bifidus, Lacto-
bacillus Insufficiency Quiz
Lactobacillus Insufficiency Quiz,
176, 177
Lactose intolerance, 200
Leg cramps, 25, 47, 97, 99, 122
Leukemia, 205
Liver disease, 24, 65, 79, 92, 95,
105, 113, 159, 207, 233, 268,
272, 275, 276, 282
Liver Dysfunction Syndrome, 275-
280
Liver spots, 73, 92, 136, 153, 187,
239, 243; *see also* Age spots,
Brown spots
Low blood pressure, 26, 40, 46,
131, 144, 252

M

MSG 11, 18, 47, 64, 71, 163, 183,
203, 220-224
Macular degeneration, 32, 33, 50,
80, 92, 104, 137, 149, 241
Magnesium, 3, 12, 15, 38, 42, 67,
109, 116-123, 142, 173, 174,
204, 207
Malabsorption Syndrome, 282-285
Manganese, 14, 15, 123-126
Mania, 45, 47, 49, 52, 170, 213,
243, 251, 256, 262, 266, 287
Margarine. *See* Hydogenated fats/
oils, Hydrogenated Fats Quiz
Megaloblastic anemia, 50; *see also*
Pernicious anemia
Melanoma, 47, 48, 89
Memory loss, 5, 23, 24, 35, 36,
40, 48, 52, 55, 114, 131, 170,
208, 212, 223, 246, 260, 289-90
Menstrual cramps, 111, 118, 172,
264, 272
Menstrual cycle, 44, 119, 149
Minerals, 2, 9-16, 42, 116, 126,
143, 154, 193, 196-198, 204,
207, 208, 255, 275, 285, 287,
289; *see also* individual minerals
Monosodium glutamate. *See* MSG

N

Nausea, 26, 40, 46, 59, 119, 144,
204, 260, 268
Nervousness, 25, 28, 31, 40, 44,
46, 49, 55, 97, 99, 101, 119,
132, 152, 156, 170, 172, 208,
223, 224, 232-235, 246, 252
Niacin, 22, 34-37, 109, 193, 224,
249, 250
Night blindness, 77, 80
Night sweats, 118, 268, 272
Nightmares, 26, 219, 260
Nitrated Meats Quiz, 228-231
Nitrates, 64, 91, 183, 228-231,
239, 241, 242
Nitrites, 228, 230, 231
Nitrosamines, 228-231
Noise sensitivity, 26, 40, 253
Nosebleeds, 73, 85, 89, 95, 97,
159, 161, 176
Numbness, 25, 56, 100, 107, 128;
see also Parasthesia.
Nutrients. *See* individual nutrients

O

Obesity, 7, 103-105, 167, 169,
172, 196, 208, 222
Oils, 11, 71, 76, 77, 79-81, 89-92,
168-171, 173, 174, 183, 184,
187, 192, 239, 242, 244, 273,
277, 279; *see also* Hydrogenated
fats/oils, Hydrogenated Fats
Quiz, Fish oils, Fats, Essential
fatty acids
Osteoporosis, 79, 81, 83, 85, 87,
96, 98, 119, 128, 139, 140, 150,
242, 281

Ovarian cysts, 172, 247, 272

P

PABA, 152, 153, 243
Pancreatitis, 24, 137, 156, 164
Panic attacks, 40, 156, 253, 260
Pantothenic acid, 2, 3, 12, 22, 37, 39, 41, 42, 109, 144, 145, 187, 212, 213, 216, 231, 234, 235, 242, 243, 251, 255-257, 274, 287
Paranoia, 5, 25, 52, 55, 144, 252, 260
Parasites, 18, 176, 267-271, 277, 274
Parkinson's disease, 7, 88, 93, 98, 116, 121, 172, 184, 191, 208
Paronychia, 146
Pasta Quiz, 197-198
Pau D'arco, 266, 267
Pellagra, 5, 7, 22, 34
Petechiae, 73, 95, 160, 161
Phosphorus, 86, 127
Pityriasis, 86
PMS, 48, 50, 118, 120, 172, 212, 216, 234, 246, 253, 272; see also Menstrual cramps
Pneumonia, 17, 110, 111, 146, 159, 216
Polycythemia, 206
Potassium, 2, 12, 14, 15, 109, 117, 130-133, 142, 213, 243, 248, 251, 256, 258
Primrose oil, 173, 174, 180, 188, 192, 266
Protein, 2, 5, 7, 10, 11, 25, 29, 42-44, 46, 47, 49, 53, 56, 58, 59, 77, 101, 102, 115, 117, 125, 127, 134, 144, 147, 149, 151, 154, 155, 157, 162-65, 169, 201, 202, 208, 216, 221, 245, 255, 261, 262, 275; see also Amino acids.

Protozoans, 267
Psoriasis, 7, 40, 81, 85, 139, 110, 164, 169, 171, 176, 184, 192, 242, 264, 283
Psychosis, 5, 24, 47, 49, 52
Pycnogenol, 160, 161, 187-189, 242-244
Pyorrhea, 50, 52, 128, 167, 216; see also Gum disease, Gums
Pyridoxine, 22, 43-49, 216, 243, 287; see also Vitamin B-6

R

Radiation, 8, 53, 64, 82, 88, 90, 91, 93, 134, 135, 137, 153, 159; see also X-rays
Rashes, 110, 149, 152, 201, 225-227, 253
Receding gums, 40, 167, 239
Recipes, 301-307
Refined Milk Products quiz, 198-200
Refined Sugar Quiz, 207-213
Refined Sugar-in-Beverage Quiz, 214-216
Restless leg syndrome, 40, 118, 122
Retardation, 45, 170
Rice polishings, 27, 28, 35-37, 60, 103-105, 125-127, 129, 213, 235, 236, 256-258, 261
Rickets, 4, 5, 7
Royal jelly, 39, 41, 42

S

Salt, 38, 108, 110, 112, 141-145, 179, 245, 248, 253, 255, 256, 261; see also Sodium
Schizophrenia, 36, 45, 47, 52, 208
Sciatica, 45
Scleroderma, 17, 140, 184
Scurvy, 4, 5, 7, 62, 286

Seizures, 85, 143, 170, 179, 219
Selenium, 3, 6, 12, 15, 42, 67, 133-138, 187, 188, 192, 213, 216, 223, 224, 227-231, 234, 236, 242, 243, 250, 251, 256, 257, 265, 266, 271, 278, 280, 287
Serotonin, 44, 49
Shingles, 41, 161
Shortness of breath, 25, 55, 115, 168, 225, 227
Silicon, 138-141, 204
Sjogren's syndrome, 170, 172
Skin, 14, 20, 26, 27, 31, 33-35, 47, 58, 59, 62, 73, 75, 77-79, 81, 82, 85, 89, 92, 95, 98, 106, 111, 115, 136, 138, 139, 147-149, 152-154, 156, 160, 167, 171, 174, 178, 179, 187, 204, 212, 239, 240, 242-244, 246, 247, 263-265, 269, 282, 283, 290
Sleep apnea, 25, 41, 122
Sleep walking, 26
Sluggish Thyroid Syndrome, 245-250
Sodium, 2, 111, 137, 141-145, 252; *see also* Salt, Sea Salt, Sodium Wasting Syndrome
Sodium Wasting Syndrome, 141-143
Spirulina, 57, 155, 157, 279, 280
Spleen, 61, 77, 113, 204, 263
Sprains, 107, 125, 146, 241
Sties, 75, 148
Steroids, 65, 258, 265, 276; *see also* Cortisone
Stretch marks, 148
Stroke, 6, 7, 67, 96, 121, 130, 132, 142, 161, 208, 242, 275
Sugar, 10, 11, 15, 18, 19, 23, 25-27, 29, 32, 33, 36-38, 41, 42, 53, 54, 57-61, 64-71, 75, 79, 91, 99-107, 117-119, 121, 124, 125, 128, 129, 131, 132, 138, 140, 143, 145, 147-151, 154, 155, 157, 162-165, 169, 172, 173, 183, 197, 200, 204, 207-216, 225, 239, 241, 242, 244, 248, 249, 251, 252, 254-262, 264, 265, 273, 276-279, 282, 287, 290
Sulfites, 11, 12, 64, 162, 183, 204, 225-228
Sunlight, 63, 78, 81, 84, 86, 87, 89, 98, 99, 137, 152, 240, 241
Superoxide dismutase, 106, 242, 244, 276
Sweating, 2, 26, 40, 118, 225, 246, 252, 260, 268, 272

T
Taste, 56, 78, 107, 142, 143, 145, 148, 194, 241, 255, 287, 290
Tea, 24, 26, 27, 42, 64, 65, 72, 115, 120, 121, 179, 180, 215, 226, 233, 257
Thiamine, 5, 12, 22-29, 109, 193, 223, 224, 236, 243, 249, 250, 261, 262, 276, 279, 280
Thymus, 61, 77, 221
Thyroid gland, 61, 77, 109, 110, 120, 129, 166, 213, 245, 249, 250, 263
Thyroid hormone, 45, 108, 110, 129, 248, 250, 276
Thyroiditis, 153
Tongue, 30-32, 35, 36, 46, 52, 55, 114, 148, 225, 282
Tooth decay, 47, 85, 216
Toothaches, 128
Tremors, 99, 100, 128, 131, 234, 235, 240, 259
Tropical sprue, 50; *see also* Malabsorption Syndrome
Tryptophan, 33, 44

326

Tyrosine, 109, 213, 224, 235, 236, 248-250, 255-257

U-V

Ulcerative colitis, 50, 56, 95, 117, 122, 130, 153, 176, 177, 234, 265, 283

Ulcers, 32, 78, 80, 146, 159, 161, 268

Vaginitis, 202

Vanilla bean, 18, 42, 232-234

Varicose veins, 92, 96, 139, 160, 179, 240

Vitamin A, 11, 67, 76-79, 99, 225, 228, 231, 242, 251, 256, 257, 265, 266, 274, 285, 287; *see also* Beta carotene

Vitamin B-1, 12, 20, 22-29; *see also* Thiamine

Vitamin B-2. *See* Riboflavin

Vitamin B-3. *See* Niacin

Vitamin B-5. *See* Pantothenic acid

Vitamin B-6, 3, 12, 42-49, 157, 158, 165, 173, 174, 188, 193, 224, 231, 234, 235, 249, 250, 257, 265-267, 274, 284, 285

Vitamin B-12, 5, 52, 54-58, 227, 228

Vitamin D, 81-87, 98, 99-101, 126, 127, 129, 288

Vitamin E, 6, 11, 12, 67, 88-94, 137, 138, 160, 162, 167-169, 174, 187-189, 191, 192, 223-225, 229, 231-233, 242, 243, 251, 256, 257, 265, 266, 274, 279, 280, 285, 288

Vitamin K, 82, 94-96

Vitiligo, 152, 153, 239

W

Water Deficiency (Dehydration) Quiz, 178-180

Weight loss, 14, 55, 58, 59, 78, 156, 168, 172, 204, 215, 268, 282

White blood cells, 61, 110, 134

White Flour Quiz, 193-197

Wild game, 139, 141

Wound healing, 31, 51, 73, 85, 107, 136, 139, 148, 156, 167, 171

X-Z

X-rays, 64, 74, 90-92, 109, 110, 134, 153

Yeast-in-Foods Quiz, 201-203

Yeast/Fungus Syndrome, 262-267

Zinc, 3, 12, 14, 15, 105-107, 109, 146-151, 157, 158, 165, 173, 174, 188, 205, 207, 216, 231, 248-251, 261, 262, 266, 271, 281, 284, 287

Dr. Igram's Books

#1 *Eat Right to Live Long* — $18.95
300 pages   6 x 9 inch softbound   ISBN 0911119221

Dr. Igram's most comprehensive book on diet and nutrition. Describes the treatment of a wide range of illnesses through diet and nutritional supplementation. Emphasis is on the nutritional treatment of heart disease, high cholesterol, high triglycerides, diabetes, obesity, allergic illnesses, arthritis, and alcoholism. Step-by-step nutritional protocols, dietary instruction, and 100 recipes included.

#2 *Self-Test Nutrition Guide* — $29.95
330 pages   5½ x 8½ inch hardbound   ISBN 0911119515

Test yourself to determine your nutritional deficiencies *from A to zinc*. Other tests show evidence of possible health problems such as adrenal insufficiency, chemical toxicity, thyroid insufficiency, intestinal malabsorption, liver dysfunction, and premature aging. Sugar, caffeine, sulfite, food dye, and MSG overload also evaluated. Each test followed by specific nutritional recommendations.

#3 *Who Needs Headaches?* — $13.95
164 pages   6 x 9 inch softbound   ISBN 0911119329

A nutritional approach to solving the migraine dilemma. Emphasizes food allergies, nutritional deficiencies, and hormonal disturbances and how to diagnose what to do about it. Chapter on structural therapy for tension headaches included.

#4 *Killed on Contact: The Tea Tree Oil Story* — $11.95
110 pages   5½ x 8½ inch softbound   ISBN 0911119493

Some things need to be killed: bacteria, viruses, fungi, parasites, and parasitic insects. Learn how to battle infectious disease with tea tree oil, Nature's most versatile and potent antiseptic. Information particularly valuable for homemakers, travelers, wilderness buffs, fishermen, and athletes.

#5 *The Survivor's Nutritional Pharmacy: A Disaster Survival Guide* —
$11.95 - 137 pages   5½ x 8½ inch softbound   ISBN 0911119442

Natural disasters, toxic waste spills, fires, parasite infestations, accidents, radiation leakage, and water contamination all demand immediate action. Learn to deal with both major and minor disasters using only natural remedies which are both safe and effective. Destroy ticks, stop wound infection, end the pain of toothache, neutralize animal/insect bites, abort diarrhea and/or dysentery, treat burns/cuts—all with natural substances.

Dr. Igram's Cassette Tape Series

#1 *How to Eat Right Series* — $39.95
   3 Tapes   Total time: 3 hours

Includes tapes on the following subjects: *How to Eat Right at Home, while Traveling, or in Restaurants; Disease Prevention; Is Our Water Safe?;* and *Preventing Aging.*

#2 *Disaster Survival Series* — $29.95
   3 Tapes   Total time: 1 1/2 hours

Please see the following page for ordering instructions for Dr. Igram's books and cassette tape series.

Order Form

Item	Quantity	Amount
A. Book #1 *Eat Right to Live Long*	_____	_____
B. Book #2 *Self-Test Nutrition Guide*	_____	_____
C. Book #3 *Who Needs Headaches?*	_____	_____
D. Book #4 *Killed on Contact*	_____	_____
E. Book #5 *The Survivor's Nutritional Pharmacy:* *A Disaster Survival Guide*	_____	_____
F. Cassette #1 *How to Eat Right Series*	_____	_____
G. Cassette #2 *Disaster Survival Series*	_____	_____

Sub-Total	_____
Sales Tax (if any)	_____
Shipping*	_____
TOTAL	_____

* *Shipping Charges:* $3.50 for single book orders - add .50¢ for each additional book. Cassette tape series (no book orders): $4.00. Payment by check, money order, or credit card.

Make checks payable to: AICM
212 Willow Parkway
Buffalo Grove, Illinois 60089
Phone: (800) 243-5242

For VISA/Mastercard orders provide the following information:

Card # _____ Exp. Date _____

Signature _____

Name _____

Address _____

City _____ State _____ Zip _____